THE
HISTORY
OF
AMERICAN
NURSING

Edited by
Susan Reverby, Wellesley College

A GARLAND SERIES

EDUCATIONAL STANDARDS FOR NURSES

with Other Addresses on Nursing Subjects

Isabel Hampton Robb

GARLAND PUBLISHING, INC.
NEW YORK • LONDON
1985

For a complete list of the titles in this series see the final pages of this volume.

This facsimile was made from a copy in the library of the University of Pennsylvania.

Library of Congress Cataloging in Publication Data

Robb, Isabel Hampton, 1859-1910.
 Educational standards for nurses.

 (The History of American nursing)
 Reprint. Originally published: Cleveland : Koeckert, 1907.
 Includes bibliographical references.
 1. Nursing—Study and teaching—Standards—United States. 2. Nursing—Standards—United States. I. Title. II. Series. [DNLM: 1. Education, Nursing—standards—United States. WY 18 R631e 1907a]
RT79.R6 1985   610.73′071173   85-4419
ISBN 0-8240-6522-0 (alk. paper)

The volumes in this series are printed on acid-free, 250-year-life paper.

Printed in the United States of America

EDUCATIONAL STANDARDS FOR NURSES.

EDUCATIONAL STANDARDS FOR NURSES

WITH OTHER ADDRESSES ON NURSING SUBJECTS

BY

ISABEL HAMPTON ROBB,

LATE PRINCIPAL OF JOHNS HOPKINS HOSPITAL
TRAINING SCHOOL FOR NURSES

E. C. KOECKERT
715 Rose Building
CLEVELAND
1907 .

CONTENTS

NOTE.

In response to many requests, I have brought together in book form several of the articles that I have written on Nursing Subjects with particular reference to those dealing with the three years' Course of training. THE AUTHUR.

I
EDUCATIONAL STANDARDS FOR NURSES.

I

EDUCATIONAL STANDARDS FOR NURSES.*

WHILE fully appreciating the honor done me by our Chairman, it has not been without much hesitancy that I have undertaken to express my views upon so important and complex a subject as "The standards of education for nurses." The subject is important because it deals with the problems of health and disease, of life and death. It is complex because so many diverse factors and interests must be taken into consideration. The social problems of human misery and suffering and how best to alleviate them have been wonderfully worked out since the days when Charles Dickens first began to exert the power of his genius upon the mind of the public in order to bring it to an active sense of its responsibility in such matters, and perhaps in no branch of philanthropy has the change been so marked as in the care of the sick of all classes in all countries. And when we consider the few years which have elapsed since the modern system of nursing has been introduced, and contrast the present

* International Congress of Charities, Correction and Philanthropy. Section III, Chicago, 1893.

conditions with those which formerly prevailed, we might at first sight perhaps be excused if we regarded our present methods with some complacency instead of all the time struggling to find room or ground for improvement. But with progress going on in every branch around us, are we alone to stand still?

The present history of hospitals in America shows that the hospital nursing is with few exceptions already being done by the members of regularly organized schools for nurses, and that where such schools do not exist steps are being taken for establishing them. Next, we find that the demand for trained nurses is steadily on the increase for cases of sickness in private families, and what is still more important, that district nursing is being introduced into almost every large city in the country. Then, too, missionary boards are requiring that their women for foreign work shall prepare themselves by receiving a course of training in nursing. Lastly, when we see that women are beginning to look upon a thorough knowledge of nursing as an essential ground work for their medical education, we cannot but be convinced that training schools for nurses and trained nurses are established facts—important factors in hospitals, in homes and for the community at large.

In considering the standard of education requisite for such workers we have to consider (1) the kind and quality of the work required, and (2) the order of woman necessary to meet such requirements.

In the daily routine of a hospital, with its variety of patients, the work of a nurse, even while herself receiving instruction, is not without its immediate results. The hospital is her workshop in which she must serve an apprenticeship, and from the day she enters it the preservation of human life and the alleviation of human suffering are to some extent delivered into her hands. Can a woman, in any other kind of work which she may choose for herself, find a higher ideal or a graver responsibility? Where human life and health are concerned, what shall we term "the little things"?

Again, in the progress that medical science is making she has her allotted part to perform. To be sure she is only the handmaid of that great and beautiful science in whose temple she may only serve in minor parts, but none the less is it her duty to endeavor to grasp the import of its teachings, that she may fulfil wisely her share. It requires, for instance, more than mechanical skill on the part of a nurse to follow the preparations for an antiseptic operation, full of significance as it is in every detail, and the saying that "dust is danger" must have a bacteriologically practical application in her mind. Nor can just any one appreciate the full meaning of the physician when he says "the nursing will be half the battle in this case.'' For the simple performance of nursing work such knowledge is requisite, but when the wider duties of either head-nurse in a hospital or principal of a school for nurses are assumed, where one must not only know, but be capable of imparting that knowledge to others, then the responsibilities become proportionately greater.

Turning from hospitals to consider the requirements for this work elsewhere, we find that nursing in private families and district nursing among the poor in their homes are the two great fields in which the nurse will be principally occupied. Here she is frequently even more closely identified as the physician's lieutenant, for whereas in a hospital a doctor is usually within ready call to render either advice or assistance, on the other hand in private practice her knowledge and skill in the absence of the physician must be depended upon in critical illnesses or unlooked-for complications until his aid may be secured. To this part of the work in particular may be applied the following words taken from a physician's address dealing with the relation of the nurse's work to that of the physician: ''The hands of a nurse are the physician's hands lengthened out to minister to the sick. Her watchful presence at the bedside is a trained vigilance supplementing and perfecting his watchful care; her knowledge of his patient's condition an essential element in the diagnosis of disease; her management of the patient, the practical side of medical science. If she fails to appreciate her duties, the physician fails in the same degree to bring aid to his patient.''

In district nursing we are canfronted with conditions which require the highest order of work, but the actual nursing of the patient is the least part of what her work and influence should be among the class which the nurse will meet with. To this branch of nursing no more appropriate name can be given than ''instructive nursing,'' for educational in the best sense of the word it should be.

Realizing, then, the kind and quality of the work to be done, we pass on to the consideration of the order of woman required to perform such duties, and those of us who have had much experience with nurses, and know all we would have them to be, and how much they really must be, as the various classes of women pass in review before our mental vision, will be inclined to agree with the writer of a letter which came to me a short time since. After asking me to recommend a head-nurse for a hospital, and enumerating at length the qualities she must possess to be successful, he concluded with the words, ''In short, we require an intelligent saint.'' The idea still prevails in many minds that almost any kind of a woman will do to nurse the sick, and that the woman who has made a failure of life in every other particular may as a last resource undertake this work. After many years of continuous work among patients and nurses, I am convinced that a woman, to become a trained nurse, should have exceptional qualifications. She must be strong mentally, morally, and physically, and to do thorough work she must have infinite tact, which is another name for common-sense. She should be as one of the women of the Queen's Gardens in Ruskin's *Sesame and Lilies*, or such an one as Olive Schriner describes when she says, "A woman who does woman's work needs a many-sided, multiform culture; the heights and depths of human life must not be beyond her vision; she must have knowledge of men and things in many states, a wide catholicity of sympathy, the strength that springs from knowledge and the magnanimity that springs from strength." Only in so far as the women of our training schools attain to this standard will the institutions and communities in which they labor feel and show forth the influence of that "sweet ordering, arrangement and decision" that are woman's chief prerogatives. What class of women have the same practical privileges of learning the means to be used for the prevention of disease or of realizing their importance? Who then is so competent or who has greater opportunities for daily practising these than herself, and teaching them to others? And intelligent she ought and must be to do this wisely; otherwise she is a mere machine, performing mechanically the task before her, not knowing why or caring for what it all means, and the public loses thereby the services of one who should be valuable in showing them something at least of the beauty of the laws of hygiene and their application, and who can fortify her teaching with scientific facts.

Let us then consider (1) what is the present standard for the trained nurse, (2) what are her educational advantages, and (3) in what ways is she deficient?

The object of schools for nurses is primarily to secure to the hospital a fairly reliable corps of nurses; and it is in order to insure a continuous source of supply that such schools are established and certain inducements are offered to women to become pupils in them. These inducements are set forth in the circulars of general information published by each school. But when one compares these circulars, the teaching methods of no two schools will be found to be alike, all varying according to the demands of the various institutions and their several authorities. Each school is a law unto itself. Nothing in the way of unity of ideas or of general principles to govern all exists, and no effort towards establishing and maintaining a general standard for all has ever been attempted. Some institutions consider that a two years course of instruction is essential; others place it at a year and a half; and others again at a year. In England a few schools insist upon three years. The hours of daily work also differ widely, some requiring from their pupils nine hours a day of active service; others as high as twelve and thirteen hours. The theoretical instruction is usually not included in the nine hours work, and it is difficult to speak definitely upon this subject, as the length of such a course, the subjects and the extent to which they are taught are again dependent upon the opinion upon this matter of the governing body of each particular school. We also find no general rule governing the special attainments or degree of education required from the women who present themselves as candidates. On the contrary, a woman who has been refused by or dismissed from one school for lack of education, dishonorable conduct, inefficiency, etc., frequently gains admittance into another, where the authorities have not so high, if any, standard required from those whom they accept. But notwithstanding all these differences, each woman who graduates from any of these schools usually has a document with the high-sounding name of diploma presented to her, and henceforth she is known as a "trained nurse," which in nowise indicates what amount of knowledge or fitness she really does bring to her work. In fact it is no unusual occurrence for schools to graduate nurses whom they at once, when relieved from their presence in the hospital, refuse to recommend or sustain in their work.

A "trained nurse" may mean then anything, everything, or next to nothing, and with this state of affairs the results are far from what they should be, and public criticism is frequently justly severe upon our shortcomings, or else is content with superficiality where like meets like. This criticism falls both upon the woman herself and upon the institution which she represents. Sometimes the one only, in others both deserve censure. Can a woman be expected to give properly a hypodermic injection to a patient if her school has never taught her how this is to be done? The school and not the nurse is to be blamed for her ignorance in such a case. Or again, abscesses may follow such injections unless the nurse has been taught the practical significance of antisepsis. Or again, can she be expected to have at her fingers' ends the principles and practice of invalid dietary when she has never been practicaly taught such a thing? And when a really capable woman realizes that she does not know enough to do her work sufficiently well to honorably receive the full compensation of a skilled nurse, and that she is not worthy of such responsibility, and if she is willing to give up more time and labor to go once more into a hospital where she may be really taught what she wants to know, where shall we find one capable school!

willing to take her ? For we wish to mould our own
fresh material, not being Michael Angelos to make
Davids out of others' failures. Sadly frequent, too,
are these requests made to the authorities of our
larger schools, and in most instances they are the
fruits of the systems prevailing in our smaller hospitals and sanatoriums. Such places are legitimate
enough in their way, and indeed many are very necessary, still the mere fact that they are hospitals in
nowise justifies them in establishing training schools
for the sake of economy, and accepting as their pupils women who, perfectly ignorant of what they
need, go to them and give up a year or two years of
precious time, and then find that their education has
been thoroughly inadequate to enable them to fulfil
what is afterwards required of them. We cannot
but feel that a real injustice is often done in such
cases. If the nurse had gone into such a hospital
as a philanthropist it would be different, but she
went there for the purpose of acquiring a certain
kind of education. Again, these small hospitals, not
having the same number to select from as the larger
schools, are apt, and in fact do take women who, not
being intellectually capable of comprehending the
high calling into which they have been admitted, tend
to lower the standard to which we are striving to attain. As an instance of such small hospitals which
have come to my notice while writing on this sub-

ject, I have in my mind one, the superintendent of which informed me that their hospital contained 30 beds and that they had a training school of 11 nurses. But the most pernicious of small hospitals is the specialty hospital or private sanatorium, which owes its existence solely to the desire of the owner to make money for himself, and in which a training school is organized for the sake of securing cheap nursing, with an utter disregard for the interests of the women employed. One doctor who owns such a hospital with 25 beds has 16 nurses, who are given a two years' course in this particular specialty, but four of these nurses are actually sent to his private patients at $25 per week, this money going to the hospital, while the nurse receives $16 per month.

This brings us to the question of the advisability of sending nurses out of the hospital into families during the second year of their training. It is true that such a procedure materially assists in the maintenance of the hospital, and to some institutions it is very necessary, but is it exactly what should be done in the best interests of the education of the nurse? The majority of schools make the statement in their general circular that they reserve the right to send their pupils out to private duty during their second year, in order to help to meet the expense of their maintenance and education. This may have been all well and good in the earlier schools when hospitals were not so numerous in the land and when the question of supporting them was a more serious difficulty than now. The additional expense of maintaining a school was not to be thought of, and it was thus necessary to appropriate some of the pupils' time towards providing an income. But now that wealthy philanthropists and societies are erecting hospitals of all kinds, they should see to it that the question of maintaining a nursing corps is provided for, instead of expecting the nurses to do philanthropic work by earning money to support the hospital at the sacrifice of their own education. As a matter of fact the services rendered by a good training school to a hospital are sufficient to warrant the expenses incurred by the school, for in any case a certain amount of work has to be performed, and for those who do it the hospital would be obliged to provide board and lodging or the equivalent in money besides the regular wages. Under what other system then could an equally efficient class of workers be secured in the same systematic way, giving a full nine hours service daily and receiving financially less than the ward maids? It is understood that the equivalent is to be made up by the education given. Is it not then a most serious responsibility on the part of such hospitals or training schools to see that the education is made as complete as possible?

After much practical experience, I maintain that

no such course of education can be thoroughly given in one year, but yet I find that very many schools limit their didactic teaching to the first year and make the second year's work of a purely practical nature and divide it between hospital work and private duty. It is absolutely necessary that class work and lectures should be carried on through the second year as well, and if this is done, then private nursing outside of the hospital is out of the question, as such interruptions would seriously interfere with any systematic teaching. I also hold that it is necessary to have the pupil under the daily observation and criticism of her teachers. This is impossible if she leaves the hospital for private duty, and one of two things must be true, viz: either she is as yet unfit to be entrusted to do her work without some supervision, or else, if she is really capable of doing this work in the second year she should not be held by the school at all. In the latter case, why not make the term of pupilage only one year and graduate her? There is another side to this question, that of justice to the patient, but as this does not really come under the head of the standards we are just now discussing we will pass it by.

It may seem that I find little that is good in the system at present followed in our training schools. I am far from wishing to disparage pioneer efforts, but I would maintain that now that our oldest school in America has attained to its majority, we can no longer fall back upon the plea that our art is still in its infancy. Our founders achieved well and nobly, but it surely was not intended that we should work on forever on the old lines. There are plenty of problems to work out, and schools for nurses are capable of much finer work than has yet been done, if we to whose hands the work is now entrusted are willing to take a broad and comprehensive view of the subject. The principal of a school for nurses performs the least part of her duty, and throws away many of her priviliges, if she is content to confine herself to the limitations of her own particular school. She must look into and go abroad among other schools, and teach her nurses to do the same, recognizing what is good in others and being ever ready to adopt any improvement. There is so much that we can learn from each other, and sooner or later we must also recognize the fact that we are all trained nurses, and that until something of a common standard is reached the imperfections of the few must be borne by all. Briefly, then, some of our chief aims should be to bring about a spirit of unity among the various schools, and to establish a standard of education upon which we may all be judged. This of necessity must be based upon the opinions of no individual mind or committee, but upon the concensus of the impartial judgments of many really experienced in the requirements for such work; for in this way alone can we command a thoroughness of work and a selection of women that we cannot now boast of. In doing this, the first step should be to bring about in all our schools, as far as possible, a uniform system of instruction, so that the requirements for graduation should be about the same in each. We might well lengthen the course of instruction in training schools to three years, with eight hours a day of practical work. This would relieve the hospital and school of having to deal with so much new material at so frequent intervals. It would then be possible to select our nurses much more carefully than can sometimes be done, for it happens at times that vacancies occur which must be filled without waiting for the right candidates to present themselves, and it would insure far better results by securing to the hospital nurses with more practical experience.

A school naturally divides itself into two classes, the quite competent and those who are fairly competent. The first division is apt, bright, intelligent, and readily taught, and at the end of the second year one is unwilling to part with them just yet, seeing in them the superintendents and good hospital workers of the future, to whom the opportunity should be given of developing their executive ability. Then the incompetent ones are dull and slow of comprehension, and they require to be taught over and over again, and at the end of two years glimmerings of the fact that they are beginning to be really interested in the work for the work's sake may be discovered, and one is very loth to let them go until the interest becomes a reality, and so for them really the third year is needed before they may be safely trusted to their own devices.

The three years' course would also tend to exclude the purely commercial woman, who enters the school, and gets through the course with as little exertion to herself as possible, only seeing in everything she does future dollars and cents, and never working for the love of her work. With this length of course it would be possible to make a better subdivision of the pupils into classes, so that every member could receive her practical teaching, her class teaching and lectures according to her grade in the school and her individual ability. There should be stated times for entrance into the school, and the teaching year should be divided according to the academic terms usually adopted in our public schools and colleges. To compel a class of students to attempt to listen to a lecture on a hot July night is barbarous. The summer months should be reserved for vacations and practical nursing only. In short, the educational atmosphere should be encouraged and developed in every way possible. Even the name of ''Nurses'

Home'' should be changed to ''Nurses' School,'' as the accepted term ''Home,'' as applied to institutions, has no educational significance. And the title of the teacher should be Principal of the School, as well as Superintendent of Nurses. In this third year those who are capable should be made head-nurses, or some direct responsibility should be laid upon them, and those who wish to fit themselves for teachers in other schools should have the opportunity of acting as assistants to the principal of the school, to learn the clerical and administrative duties of such positions. In this way a class of two might be under her instruction for a year at a time, their positions being those of senior and junior assistants, with a moderate salary attached. Unfortunately, few women get these opportunities, and the majority are forced to assume the charge of training schools with no equipment for the work further than that they have been able to acquire as head-nurses; and the hospital, school, and often the new superintendent herself suffer accordingly while she is gaining the necessary experience. In fact a Normal School for preparing women for such posts is quite as necessary as those established for other kinds of teachers.

The eight-hour system will also be advisable, for the reasons that the health of the nurses will not bear the strain of a three years' course with longer hours; besides, is it not poor economy and mistaken judgment for a country to sacrifice the health of one class of people in trying to restore that of others?

Then it would do away with the continual breaks in the day's work caused by the half-day and two hours recreation system, and if a systematical course of theoretical teaching is entered upon, shorter hours of practical work are absolutely necessary, as the overpowering physical weariness following a long day's work makes mental effort out of the question, and to require tired-out women to attend evening lectures after nine hours of physical exertion, and the mental excitement attendant upon hospital work, is little short of tyranny. And this mental development is necessary for the best results in the work if we would command the services of an intelligent class of women.

In considering standards of education for nurses we must not overlook the smaller hospitals, cottage hospitals, etc., for they have their work to do as well as the large institutions, but that they are in no position to offer adequate teaching or experience to a woman who would become a thorough nurse is very evident.

How then can we meet the problem of supplying good nursing and at the same time making good nurses? It can only be met by the larger schools entering into arrangements with the smaller schools to supplement their teaching. This plan, of course, would require that the standard of women and of education should be the same, and the teaching on practically the same basis, while the head-nurses of the smaller schools must be thoroughly competent women. In a city where distances are not too great, one school may successfully undertake the care of two or three hospitals. For instance, a children's hospital may better be associated with a general training school, and the same holds good with a hospital dealing with obstetrics, or with any other special branch. As for private sanatoriums owned by private individuals, the nursing should unquestionably be done by salaried nurses who have graduated from some reputable school.

A final word as to the practical qualifications which should be required of women who present themselves as candidates to be taught nursing. A good practical English education should be insisted upon. By this is meant that the candidate should come up to the standard required to pass the final examinations in the best high schools in the country, special stress being laid upon her ability to express herself either in writing or orally with quickness and accuracy. Her knowledge of arithmetic should be of an eminently practical nature and so that she can readily deal with problems involving fractions, percentage, bookkeeping, etc. This much is absolutely necessary. Of course more than this is desirable, as no other study develops the reasoning powers in the same practical way, and women who do not possess any education in arithmetic beyond the few simple rules, simply applied, are at once placed in a disadvantageous position upon entering upon their work in a modern hospital. Of course, if she has in addition a knowledge of languages and a broad general reading, the candidate is all the better prepared for undertaking and obtaining success in her career as a nurse.

Aside from this mental equipment there are other qualifications of a practical nature that should be insisted upon. Every woman before entering upon hospital work should be a thoroughly trained housekeeper. Practical household economy should be a part of her *home education,* for in hospital wards the nurses are the stewards, the caretakers of the hospital property, and upon their thrift and careful ordering must depend the economical outlay of the hospital funds. I cannot dwell upon this practical household economy with too great emphasis, for experience has shown me to a painful extent how this branch of woman's work is neglected or superficially understood by so many women in all ranks of life. A total lack of or appreciation for the principles that govern such work will inevitably be followed by a deficiency in thoroughnes and system. In the nurse should be found evidences of this practical knowledge; it should be seen in the way she cares for her own room, her personal appearance, and in the order and system which attends any work to which she puts her hand, and her knowledge of the value of the articles she has to work with should be shown by the way she cares for them. But too often alas! training schools are obliged to not only teach in two short years all that pertains to nursing, but try as well to teach the first principles, at least, of domestic science, and much valuable time is spent in doing this that should really be given to nursing. When a graduate nurse goes into a private family and earns the just reproach of being extravagant and careless in the care of property, and when the details of her work are without finish, the blame should be put down to her early home training and not to her training as a nurse.

Time does not permit me to more than touch upon some of the most glaring defects in our system of nursing and to outline very briefly some changes that might be of general advantage, but I trust that sufficient has been said to arouse interest enough among hospital and training school workers to induce them to persevere in working out the problems, the solution of which will give us more united work and a more uniform standard of education for all who are to go out into the world as trained nurses; for only from institutions in which the head, the heart and the hand are trained to work together in harmony can come forth the true nurse.

II

THE AIMS OF THE JOHNS HOPKINS TRAINING SCHOOL FOR NURSES.

THE AIMS OF THE JOHNS HOPKINS TRAIN-
ING SCHOOL FOR NURSES.*

A LTHOUGH the existence of training schools for nurses is of but recent date, much that is good and practical has been written about them and, in view of all this excellent literature on the subject of nursing in its various phases, it is not befitting that our guests on this occasion should be treated to an exhaustive history of the rise and growth of Training Schools for Nurses in general. To-day then your attention is asked for a brief time to consider more particularly Schools for Nurses as they now exist in this country, and what the future outlook may be for them in some respects, and more especially for the one which it is our privilege to assist in opening to-day. Of the various professions opened to woman during the past few years, none has made more sure and rapid growth nor met with greater public favor than that of the trained nurse; while all of the various types of nurses which existed before her time still exist to a more or less degree, the trained nurse is acknowledged by both physician and patient, to be superior, for the simple reason that the world at

* Opening of the Johns Hopkins Hospital School for Nurses, 1889.

large now recognizes the fact that in this work, as in all others, technical skill can only be acquired through a systematic course of practical and theoretical study under competent teachers.

It seems strange that such a system of caring for the sick should have been adopted only within this last quarter of a century, for the need has always been as great, and the idea would seem to have been already suggested by the various orders of Sisters of Mercy, founded centuries ago, and which had proved by their deeds woman's capabilities in this direction. The delay certainly could not have been caused by any lack of willing women, for no doubt many existed in the past century, who would have responded to the demand for their services in hospitals, as gladly as the women of to-day, who offer themselves in such numbers, that the wonder grows how so many, whether desirable or otherwise, are willing to undertake a work of the grave responsibilities of which they are by no means kept in ignorance, when they have once decided to undertake the duties of a trained nurse.

Schools for nurses, it must be understood, consider little that is sentimental and much that is practical in deciding upon the fitness of a woman for nursing. While some candidates may have more natural aptitude for the work than others, there are other attributes no less important, that are required.

Training Schools aim to receive only women who are at least fairly intellectual, who are strong and enduring physically, and who morally will recognize the sacredness of the work that they are engaged in. Of their pupils, they require that they shall yield implicit obedience and loyalty to the physician, that they shall faithfully carry out his directions, and in his absence watch over the welfare of his patient, that they shall further his scientific study of disease, by intelligently fulfilling his orders, in administering medicines, taking account of the range of pulse and temperature, regulating the sanitary condition of the sick room, noting every unusual symptom in the patient, and reporting the various changes in his condition, as the patient responds or fails to respond to treatment.

Thus by night or by day a nurse must be on the alert, she must have at her command, presence of mind to meet any emergency, she must abound in tact and patience with those suffering from physical and mental disturbances, and be unwearying in her efforts for her patient's comfort. And all this and much more she must do cheerfully, being kind and sympathetic and adaptable to the varying necessities of the sick-room.

As an evidence of the success of Training Schools for Nurses we find them organized or being organized in all of the principal cities and towns, in connection with all kinds of hospitals. The one thing to be regretted in this connection is, that it is not .just that the authorities in very small hospitals, and in hospitals that are devoted to the treatment of one or two especial kinds of diseases, should receive women as pupil-nurses, permit them to profit only by the limited experience they gain in such hospitals, and then at the end of a few months, graduate them as qualified trained nurses. When such graduates go forth, and undertake not only the kind of work they are qualified for, but also other branches that they are almost entirely ignorant of, they bring unjust criticism on all who call themselves by the same name. The arrangement provides a cheap method of securing hospital nursing, but is fair neither to the women received by such institutions, nor to those who spend many more months and much greater labor in the larger hospitals, fitting themselves for the work of caring for any and all kinds of maladies.

While the usefulness of such small hospitals is recognized, and the considerations of efficacy and economy, which has lead them to the attempt to train nurses are fully appreciated, the question arises: Would it not be better if an arrangement could be made whereby one large school could do the nursing in several small hospitals?

Up to the present time the usefulness of schools

for nurses is recognized chiefly from three stand-points. They have solved the problem of how to properly care for the sick poor in our large charity hospitals and infirmaries, and have made it possible for private and church hospitals, to give their patients skilled care. The rich can also secure the same services in their homes. Moreover for women they have created a profession, which is unquestionably womanly. But thus far they have ministered chiefly to needs of the rich and the very poor.

The trained nurse is an almost unknown quantity to the poor in their homes, and the great majority of people with only moderate incomes, are still obliged to struggle through with their sick as of yore, as best they may, for the simple reason that a trained nurse is too great a luxury, which too often costs more than the modest income will permit, nor can the self-supporting nurse very often afford to render her services for less.

How to bring the services of the trained nurse into just such homes, is a problem that has caused and is causing food for serious thought in many minds. Commendable efforts have been put forth, especially in New York and Philadelphia, in this direction, but with scant success, for want of adequate support, and Training Schools have been quite unable to answer this call, that has come to them so often from physicians, to supply them with skilled nursing for these classes.

Most of our large Training Schools have had pioneer financial struggles for existence, and even up to this time the greater good they would gladly undertake, they have to withhold owing to lack of means, but they will not remain satisfied until the time has come when they will be in a position to add this branch of nursing to their course of study for pupil-nurses. In this particular, as in some others, The Johns Hopkins Hospital School for Nurses, that is just opening its doors to teach women the art of caring for the sick is unusually fortunate, for certainly never has a Training School for Nurses opened with brighter prospects.

As an essential part in the plan of a great hospital, that is so closely allied with a world-renowned university, already its name alone has made the first steps easy, for in place of being obliged to seek for women to become its pupils, candidates have come of their own accord, in numbers sufficient to allow the formation of its first class from women whose superior attainments promise well for the future success of the school.

The terms upon which a candidate will be accepted require, that she be between the age of twenty-three and thirty-five years, and can furnish satisfactory testimonials from a physician and a clergyman, that she enter upon a month of probation, and sometime during that month pass an examination in the elementary English branches. This is simply intended to test the applicant's ability, to take notes on lectures, to write legibly and accurately reports of her patients, and to read aloud well. This amount of education is indispensable for acceptance as a pupil. The pupil is required, when on duty, to wear the uniform prescribed by the institution, and is allowed a small compensation monthly, to be expended for uniform, text books and other expenses incidental to her training.

The hours for duty are from 7.30 A. M. to 7.30 P. M. with the usual time off for meals, and two hours additional for study, exercise and rest. Unless an emergency arises, the nurse is allowed an afternoon during the week, half of each Sunday, and a vacation of two weeks each year. The course of instruction will be given by means of classes, lectures and demonstrations by physicians and surgeons at the bed side and by the principal of the school and the head nurses.

The proposed plan of study is somewhat similar to that in other large schools for nurses. During the first year the pupils will be engaged in hospital work entirely, acting as assistants in the wards, and under the instruction of appointed head-nurses, being changed, from time to time, from one department of work to another. In connection with this practical work, they will receive theoretical teaching given sytematically in classes, and by means of lectures. In their second year, they are expected to know sufficient to be able to assume more direct responsibility of patients in the hospital, and to undertake the special care of patients in the private wards. In addition to this it is expected a certain portion of each pupil's second year will be devoted to district nursing, among the poor in their homes, under a competent head nurse, where it is hoped that such nurses may not only help to bring their sick back to health, but also leave behind them some good practical work and simple lessons in hygiene and right living, that may result in better health and happier homes. And more especially do we trust that her presence for good may be felt in this city, as it never yet has been felt in any city of America, in the homes of those with moderate incomes, who will be required to give in return for her services only in proportion to their means.

It is to be borne in mind that the duties of a nurse by no means cease when the crisis of an illness is past, for after this come days, or more often weeks of weary convalescence when the patient is often obliged to depend upon the nurse almost or entirely for companionship, and the latter's ingenuity is taxed to the utmost to render this time less irksome and tedious.

At such times professional lore is of little avail and most invaluable becomes the woman who in addition to her skill as a nurse, has at her command such powers of entertaining, as can only be afforded by a fund of general knowledge, familiarity with current events, a knowledge of what is going on in the world of art, literature and even science and a readiness to comprehend all or anything that may be of interest to her patient.

We make it a cast-iron rule that a nurse shall not entertain her patients with gossip over the affairs of her last patient, or with accounts of her hospital life and experiences, be she ever so urgently entreated to do so. But out of the fulness of the heart, the mouth giveth speech, and unless some means are provided against knowing nothing but hospital life and sick-rooms, the rut is inevitable. That this condition may be provided against, we trust that in these rooms some bright, pleasant, social hours may be passed, and among the books, magazines and papers that are sure to find their way here, when the need for them is realized, the pupils may spend valuable hours keeping bright what is already theirs and adding what is best from all, in this way storing the mind with knowledge, which shall serve as an antidote for weariness in the future days of convalescence. Thus it shall be the sincere endeavor to afford to each woman who becomes a pupil, opportunity to make herself familiar with all things that tend to perfect her as a nurse.

It is not so much the great amount of work that she can accomplish practically that is desired, but the kind of work, and that she render unto each patient under her care nursing in its best methods, and truest sense. And as the University and Hospital are looked to from all quarters for what is best in science, so may it follow, that, as time goes on and women go forth as graduates of the Johns Hopkins Hospital School for Nurses, this School may be looked to for what is best in nursing, and her graduates uphold with all faithfulness their part in a great work.

III

DISTRICT NURSING.

III

DISTRICT NURSING.*

FEW men or women can spend a number of years in hospital work, particularly in the wards of the free hospitals of large cities, without sooner or later coming to a realizing sense of the incompleteness of their work for the relief of the sick poor, whose tale of woe can be read from their condition without any words. Too often we know that this condition is the result of their daily surroundings and manner of living, and we know too that those who come under observation in hospitals are but a fraction of the whole number in the same condition. When a cure is wrought does it not seem a bit absurd, after all the time, thought and money spent upon suitable buildings and hygienic surroundings, added to all the energy and anxiety expended upon the patients, to send them out again into their former unhealthy environments, with the certainty in our hearts that some leave us only to return in a worse plight than before, and that the struggle for life must be gone all through again? Does it not seem that methods for the prevention of disease ought to

* Annual Meeting of Baltimore Charity Organization Society, 1891.

45

be more generally recognized and brought into more active use, and thus do away with the necessity for so much curative treatment?

The chief source of relief that we have to look to in such cases is the Charity Organization Society, and simple are the efforts we are asked to make. All we need do is to reach and take from a pocket a card upon which is printed the invitation, ''Send the needy to us,'' and write upon that card the name and address of the needy one, and the comfortable feeling comes that in answer to it friends will be provided who will see him through until he can do for himself. But this is quite another branch of philanthropy, with its own definite work, and does not deal directly with prevention of disease, though it nobly fulfils its part of a general plan. This will never be wholly successful until doctors, with their professional knowledge; clergymen, sisterhoods, nurses, with their trained skill, and laymen, with their wealth, time and business ability, all unite to make it so. There are numbers of sick poor for whom hospital care is utterly impossible; I would mention in particular mothers of families, the housekeepers of the homes, chronic patients, and those who still retain their old prejudices against hospitals. Their numbers are greater than you may think, and many instances might be cited that have come under our notice here in Baltimore in which the benefits of a hospital were not available.

Let us now consider what systematic means are employed for their relief, and to what extent. Until within a few years free dispensaries were considered a sufficient solution of the problem; to these are now added the Visiting Nurses' Association or District Nursing among the poor in their homes. In this country such associations are still in their infancy. In England, and particularly in London and Liverpool, the necessity for this form of nursing among the poor was recognized some years ago, and in 1868 the East London Nursing Society was founded; in 1874 another society was created, the Metropolitan and National Nursing Association. It was established after the most careful consideration, and with a standard of nursing of the highest order, and is now the leading system in Great Britain. As stated in its reports, the objects of the Association are as follows:—

1. To train and provide a body of skilled nurses to nurse the sick poor in their own homes.

2. To establish in the metropolis, and to assist in establishing in the country, district organizations for this purpose.

3. To establish a training school for district nurses in connection with one of the London hospitals.

4. To raise, by all means in its power, the standard of nursing and the social position of nurses.

In the original plan a central home and training school for nurses in district work was established, and after the work was thoroughly well under way it was increased and more patients were cared for by opening branch homes in suitable localities. In each home a competent superintendent was placed and a staff of six or more nurses given her, but as expenses increased it was found advisable to make the branch homes independent of the central one, and to have them meet their own expenses. This relieved the central home of much responsibility and expense, divided the labors, and quickened local liberality and interest. These district homes have been established in nine different parts of London. A very interesting morning spent in August 1890 at one of these district homes, Holloway, North London, enables me to speak more particularly of the work done by this one, but it is safe to say it may be taken as a criterion of the rest. The home itself is a most attractive old place; ivy-covered and standing in the midst of ample grounds, it is at once suggestive of the restful, home-like air found within. Here a superintendent and nurses reside and make daily visits within the North London district. The number of visits made by a nurse each day varies in proportion to the care required by each patient and the distance to be travelled, but the average is from eight to ten per day. The yearly statistics will give an idea of the amount they accomplish. In 1880, their first year, the number of cases nursed was 477; in 1885 they had increased to 1,257, and in 1890 to 1,700. The total number of visits made last year was 30,284. The association is supported by voluntary contributions. Patients are received from all sources, as the superintendent is in communication with physicians, the clergy, sisterhoods, Charity Organization Society, and any society working among the poor. All nursing is done strictly under medical direction. The association supplies nothing beyond the nursing and medical appliances. Necessary clothing and nourishment are provided by societies who become responsible for such supplies. Where the patients are able some slight payment is made for the nurses' services. As an evidence of the favor with which this branch of nursing is looked upon by the medical men, it is stated that more than half the number of patients sent last year were sent by them.

A decided impetus has been given district nursing in England by the contribution of a greater part of the Queen's Jubilee Fund towards this work, and plans are now under way to affiliate the Queen's Institute with societies already founded in the various cities and towns and to have a national District Association that will have its nurses, not only with the poor in the large cities, but in every town and village in the country.

It will be interesting to glance for a moment at what has been done by similar associations in the United States. They are comparatively few and of recent development, but increasing interest is being displayed in them, so it may be hoped that a few more years will find them as widely established as in England. A visit to the headquarters of the Boston Association a year ago last spring, under the kindly escort of one of the managers, enabled me to obtain some valuable information and considerable insight into their methods. The city is divided up into dispensary districts, and a trained nurse is supplied for each such district. She works under the direction of a dispensary physician, meets him at an appointed hour, gives him a report of the previous twenty-four hours, and receives directions for the day. Two managers are responsible for each district, and they receive a weekly report from the nurse. The system is simple and has succeeded admirably. The association is sustained by voluntary contributions, and up to the present has been enabled to maintain a staff of six nurses. Auxiliary relief is systematically supplied by the Loan Closet Society, the Diet Kitchen, and the New England Kitchen. An idea of the work done can be gathered from the statistics of their Fifth Annual Report. The total num-

ber of patients was 2,614; the number of visits made
by the nurses was 23,416. In this association the
nurses have no central home and no direct supervising head nurse. The organization, as its stated
Instructive District Nursing Association, as its stated
object is not only to nurse the sick, but to have the
nurse give such instruction to the women in their
homes as will enable them to take better care of themselves and neighbors, by observing the rules of whole-
some living and by practicing the simplest arts of
domestic nursing. A similar association has been, I
believe, established in Philadelphia. New York has
for some years been doing something with the work,
but not upon so broad and systematic a basis as in
the cities already mentioned. An attempt to establish
something of the kind in Chicago was made six or
eight years ago by the Felix Adler Society, but after
two or three years was dropped. Two years ago, in
the same city, the Visiting Nurses' Association was
organized and so far has met with unusual success.
It is also supported by voluntary contributions and
sustains a staff of six nurses who have fixed headquarters and a supervising head. They work in connection with relief committees. The work is to be
increased in the coming year, as the Association now
has a surplus of $2,000 on hand. In the report of
the past year the total number of patients was 1,042;
100 of these were sent to the hospital. The number

of visits made was 13,197. Indianapolis sends out nurses to sick poor from the city hospital, but beyond these cities I have not been able to learn of any others systematically engaged in this branch of philanthropy.

Nursing does not represent alone restoration to health. That might be considered as incidental in comparison with the influence exerted by these women in the homes of the poor and the preventive treatment they are able to give; for in the light of our present teaching on causation of disease by germs it is clear how necessary it is for the prevention of disease that we should put this teaching into practice. When we know that typhoid fever, diphtheria, consumption, are all the result of unhygienic conditions, should not every fresh step taken in philanthropy be in the direction of the prevention of misery and disease, by showing that cleanliness *is* next to godliness? And what better step towards accomplishing this can be taken than through some such work as this district nursing? A nurse enters the abodes of disease for an express purpose and meets the people on a common ground of interest. What better field for teaching than this constant personal contact in these homes? What opportunities to give simple object lessons in household economy. sanitation, nursing, showing that there is a healthier, better way of living, and one that helps to bring comfort and happiness!

But this highest type of nursing needs special equipment, and a nurse who succeeds in hospital or private practice would not always succeed here. In order to attain to the full scope of her work, she should have, in addition to that hospital training, the necessary tact and adaptability, and sense of the moral obligations resting upon her, the keenest knowledge of mankind; household economy should be at her finger ends and on her tongue; she should know practically how to cook, how to clean, what is wrong with the plumbing, and besides these household arts even have a knowledge of bacteriology. If she would touch the source of this great problem, her knowledge cannot be too catholic or too practical, or her object lessons too many, for she must not only tell how, but teach the reason why. It means to go down to the bottom of the darkness of ignorance and work up to the light of knowledge. Nor have we to look as far as London for a field of labor, for in our own city there are daily opportunities offered us to try what this one more way may do.

Only a few days ago a clergyman said to me: "If a choice were given me to have an assistant clergyman or a trained nurse, I should take the nurse, for daily do I meet cases where I can do nothing, but where she can do much. She would do more for me in caring for my people and helping them out of difficulties than he could;'' and this is but one instance; doctors a number of times have said, ''If only I might have a nurse to visit my patients, she would never lack for plenty of work.'' What possibilities these opportunities unfold and the pity of it that they must be lost! Although we may not have a trained nurse for each church, if only one at least might be supplied to each dispensary for a year, there is no doubt at the end of that time the annual meeting of the Charity Organization Society would have an encouraging report to present on this, to us, new branch of philanthropy.

IV

THE THREE YĔARS' COURSE OF TRAINING IN CONNECTION WITH THE EIGHT HOUR SYSTEM.

THE THREE YEARS' COURSE OF TRAINING IN CONNECTION WITH THE EIGHT HOUR SYSTEM.*

SOMETIME over a year ago it was my privilege to prepare for the International Congress of Charity and Correction a paper dealing with the standards of education to be demanded of nurses, both before and after their entrance into a training school. It may be remembered by some of you who are now present that I spoke at some length of the necessity of a careful elimination of the undesirable candidates who present themselves. I insisted that not every woman who desires to take up the profession of a trained nurse has the natural capabilities or has had the educational advantages which are necessary to such a career. But I pointed out that, after obtaining suitable material, it is necessary to make the best possible use of it, and that here the second part of our duty begins.

Among other changes advocated in the paper just referred to was the extension of the course over a

---

* Annual Convention American Society of Superintendents' of Training Schools for Nurses, Boston, 1895.

period of three years, with a day of practical work consisting of eight hours. At that time the reasons for these changes and suggestions as to the manner in which they could be carried out could be only broadly outlined. The object of the present paper is to consider these reasons in detail and try to arrive at some practical conclusion which will facilitate the establishment of such a course in the various training schools.

The subject should be dealt with without bias for any school in particular, but with a view to the best interests of all training schools which are able to undertake satisfactorily the important duty of training nurses. Between these schools there should exist a spirit of unity, and it should be our earnest desire to establish a standard of education that will be common to all. To bring about this should be, and I believe is, one of the chief aims of our association. And it seems to me that, just at present, no better opportunity could be afforded us to accomplish our end than in uniting in developing the three years' course of instruction, and agreeing, after due discussion, upon the adoption of some scheme which should also include (1) specifications of the necessary qualifications of applicants; (2) a curriculum for teaching and study, and (3) a proper grading in tests and in final examinations for certificates.

That some extension of the period of training is

generally desired was evidenced by the informal discussion of the subject that took place in this assembly last year; by the suggestions since offered by the writers in our various magazines devoted to the subject of nursing, and by the fact that since the International Congress some one or two schools have lengthened their course so as to make it extend over three years, while others have this step under serious consideration.

A superintendent of a training school owes a duty, first, to the hospital, and, secondly, to the nurses under her. These duties are of equal importance; the hospital must not be sacrificed, but neither have we any right to sacrifice the well-being of our nurses; some scheme must be adopted which shall prove advantageous to both. I shall, therefore, consider a little in detail the advantages or disadvantages to the hospital and to the nurses which may result from the adoption of the plan suggested. For the hospital the advantages are readily seen. In the first place, the hospital would have better nurses, since it would be benefitted by having more experienced nurses during the third year of their course. Again, the hospital and training school would be relieved of the disadvantages of having to deal with so much raw material at such frequent intervals, and the school would be enabled to select from the candidates much more closely, and thus a higher standard could be more easily obtained.

If the third year's instruction were made to include a course for nurses who wished to prepare themselves more especially for hospital positions, the hospital would again be benefited, because, under present conditions, superintendents of schools have no opportunity of learning the administrative duties of such a position until after they have undertaken it. Our present methods of training allow but few opportunities for a woman to gain this practical knowledge, hence the success of a new superintendent of a training school must depend upon her native ability and such stray knowledge as she may have been able to pick up while occupying the position of head nurse. More than one nurse's career as a superintendent has been cut short by mistakes through ignorance in the beginning of her administration, mistakes which would never have occurred had she had an opportunity beforehand to become practically acquainted with the duties of her new position. Again, it must not be forgotten that while such a process of development is going on, and the superintendent is becoming competent, the hospital and pupils alike suffer, and the best work and the best teachings are not attainable.

A third year is also necessary in many cases to complete the training of pupils, who, while having all the requisite qualities of goodness and reliability, are not intellectually over-bright, and need an additional year to make them thoroughly competent in their profession. Then, there are others who, while exactly opposite, are bright, quick and easily taught, nevertheless lack a thorough comprehension of the dignity and responsibility which they have undertaken, and who do not fully appreciate the value of the discipline which they receive in the course of their training. For such pupils the protection, influence and teaching of the school during an additional third year are necessary before they can be safely left to their own judgment. In any case, a third year is to be regarded as a period of assimilation or digestion, without which the learning of the first two years will be far less valuable. That many nurses feel that they are not fully qualified at the end of two years is evidenced by the number of intelligent women who love their work, and who are interested in their profession, and who beg to be allowed to stay another year. By the establishment of the three years' course it is hoped that the number of such women would be much increased, since we may naturally expect and hope that the commercial woman will be excluded by the adoption of this plan, and, even if we have fewer graduate nurses, they are much more likely to be competent, and after all this is the main point. As a matter of fact, a slight diminution in number would not be an altogether unmixed evil. Just now the number of graduate nurses engaged in private nursing is, I am told, so great, and is growing so rapidly all the time, that many nurses are without patients half the time. I am informed that in the city of Philadelphia there are so many that a committee of physicians have already held a meeting in order to discuss the possibility of taking advantage of this condition, in order to reduce the remuneration for the services of graduate nurses—a somewhat unwarrantable proceeding on their part it would seem. But if this question is to be regulated by the laws of supply and demand, then a diminution in the number of graduates will insure a lucrative occupation to those who have had a thorough training, and who hold certificates of competency.

So much for the advantage of a three years' course to the hospital and to the nurses. But should this change alone be made, we would be worse off than before, and unless the day's work of practical nursing be limited to eight hours it would be better to go on as at present. The board of trustees recognize the advantages which would accrue to the hospitals from the adoption of the three years' course, and they would cheerfuly add on the third year were it not for the fear of additional expense which would be incurred should the day's work be shortened to eight hours. I shall have some suggestions to make later on, which will perhaps relieve them to a great extent of anxiety on this point. But, first, I wish to bring forward a few reasons why one change necessarily involves the other. On the question of the length of the day's practical work, we superintendents of training schools ought to know more than other hospital authorities. We have been through every step of nursing work ourselves, and should be best competent to judge of what is right and expedient in the matter, and if we are convinced that a day of eight hours is sufficient, we should all agree in giving the project our warmest support. We are the representatives of the nurses, and if we do not advocate their rights and interests, we can hardly expect others to take thought of us.

As I said just now, a superintendent of a training school undoubtedly has obligations to the hospital in which she works, and is in duty bound to give it her best thought, work and loyalty, but she has, at the same time, obligations and responsibilities also to the nurses who put themselves under her care.

I am sure that many of you have had some qualms of conscience at the way in which we are sometimes forced, I might almost say, to drive our pupil nurses through a two years' course. I assure you that I have had myself many anxious moments for the future of certain of my pupils, more especially as regards their health. It is well known that a combination of physical and mental labor is more exhausting than simple manual or simple mental occupation. It is true that for a time such a strain can be borne without producing any permanent injurious effects, and it is possible in most cases for women to stand the strain imposed upon them for two years, although I am afraid that not all of them come out of the trial unscathed. If, however, this high pressure is to be kept up for three years, I am sure that the health of the nurses will suffer. A woman who works physically over eight hours a day is in no mental condition to profit to any extent by class instruction or lectures, and it is very questionable if a woman working ten, eleven, twelve, or more hours a day for three years will be equal to really good work during the third year, even if her health apparently holds out to the end of her time. Able-bodied laboring men are now everywhere advocating a working day consisting of eight hours. If this is a reasonable demand, then we are surely not justified by putting a harder task upon women who are not only upon their feet during the greater part of their time, but in addition have an enormous tax being constantly made upon their patience and temper, as well as being burdened with no little mental anxiety and responsibility.

From another standpoint let me ask, will the patients obtain the best nursing in this way, and is a neurasthenic nurse fit to take charge of patients?

I maintain, therefore, that the three years' course must not be considered at all unless the hours of practical work are shortened, but if the two changes can be made together, then the preservation of the health of the nurse and the extension of her education and training will be insured. This again will result in an increase in her competency, and consequently will be productive of greater benefits to the patients which come under her care during her training and after she has graduated.

I said just now that we must take into consideration certain means of meeting the extra expenses which might be incurred if the staff of nurses be increased in order that the hours of work may be shortened. I commend this problem to the ingenuity of every one of my hearers and shall be glad if the discussion evoked by this paper may bring out something better than what I myself have at the present time to propose. It seems to me that if the eight-hour system were once set in good running order, it would be found that the necessary increase in the number of nurses would be very small. The two propositions which I would submit are as follows: First, a uniform remuneration for each of the three years, instead of an increase every year, according to our present custom; second, the adoption of a three years' course, with a working day of eight hours, without remuneration.

At the present time the practice is to allow the pupil nurses eight dollars a month for the first, and twelve dollars a month for the second year. We say in our circulars that "this is in nowise intended as a salary, but is allowed for uniforms, text-books and other expenses incidental to their training." If this money is not intended as a remuneration for services rendered, why is the amount increased the second year, seeing that the expenses are in reality much greater the first year, when the probationer has to supply herself with the necessary text-books and a full set of uniforms. If the amount allowed during the first year is sufficient, then the second years' allowance is more than enough; in any case, the expenses of a third year would not be more than those of either of the other two, and the allowance need not be increased for the third year. Would it not be better to make a uniform allowance, say of ten dollars a month for all the course? The extra expense, then, to the hospital would resolve itself into the cost of maintenance of a certain number of additional nurses, together with their allowance of ten dollars a month.

The second proposition should, I think, find no objection, at least on the part of hospital trustees, and, as I shall explain later, the apparent objections

from the nurses' standpoint, are not insuperable.
This proposition advocates the establishment of a
three years' course, with a practical working day of
eight hours, on the non-payment plan. The pupils
would thus receive their uniform, board, room, laundry work and a really liberal education as an equivalent for the three years' service, as a result of which
they would be qualified for lucrative posts, either as
superintendents of training schools, managers of
small hospitals, private nurses, assistants to practicing physicians, or, in fact, to fill any position where
the knowledge and skill of a trained nurse can be
fully utilized. This non-payment system would also
place the schools, at once, on a scholastic basis, and
be another means of attracting to them as students
refined and intelligent women. In this connection,
scholarships could be founded, which would be the
means of helping poor but really competent women
to their education. I am not sure that nurses more
than any others who are preparing to enter a scientific profession should expect to be self-supporting
from the very outset, and I do not believe that this
arrangement would hinder any desirable additions to
our numbers.

But above all, such an arrangement would leave no
solid ground upon which hospital authorities could
object to the two changes just advocated, since the
requisite increase in members would add but little to

the expense, and some of the money now devoted to the remuneration of the pupil nurses could be spent in paying a traind staff of head nurses, all of which should be graduates.

Further expense could be saved by having only one responsible head under the superintendent of the hospital for domestic management. In fact, it is only by such an arrangement that the third year's training could be made as practical as it should be. This position should be occupied by the superintendent of nurses and principal of the training school, so that besides the responsibility of the work of the nurses in the wards she should have the care of the nurses' home, the linen room, the laundry, and the buying for the hospital. Her staff should consist of a graduate head nurse in each ward, one for the nurses' home, one for the laundry and linen room, and one for the office. Their assistants in all these departments should be drawn from the pupil nurses of the third year; the head nurse might also be a third year nurse. The division of the practical work during the three years might be somewhat as follows:

For the first two years—Four months in the medical wards; four months in the surgical wards; three months in the gynæcological wards; one month in obstetrics; two months in the children's wards; three months in the private wards; two months in the operating rooms, one month in the diet school; one month in the dispensary; one month on special duty; one month on vacation.

For the third year—Two months obstetrics; four months as assistant in superintendent's office; three months as assistant in laundry and linen room; three months as assistant in nurses' home.

During the six months in the superintendent's office, the assistants preparing for hospital positions would be expected to give a certain amount of class-teaching to pupils of the first and second years. Nurses preparing for private duty should spend part of their third year in the wards, but all should serve their time in the linen room, and in the performance of the housekeeping duties at the home.

The first two years' teaching would consist of classes and lectures covering about the same ground as at present. Class instruction could be given twice instead of once a week, and since the pupils would have more time and the instructors would be more numerous, the various subjects could be dealt with much more thoroughly than with our present system. For third year students, class instruction could be given once, or perhaps twice a week. The first four months of the first year could be devoted to class instruction on practical nursing and materia medica only, the second four months to human anatomy and physiology. At the end of the first year examinations might be held upon: (1) practical nursing;

(2) materia medica; (3) anatomy and physiology; (4) diet. At the end of the second year: (1) children; (2) medical nursing, including massage; examination of urine and hygiene; (3) surgical nursing, including the duties of the operating room and the nurse's duty in emergencies; (4) gynæcological and obstetrical nursing.

The third year examination should include: (1) methods to be adopted in class teaching; (2) administrative duties of the superintendents of training schools; (3) practical care of the wards, the nurses' home, linen room and laundry; (4) hospital buying and supplies; (5) private nursing.

I need not say that the above is only a suggestive sketch for the third year teaching; I have only tried to indicate the leading points. It will remain for the association to draw up a schedule in which certain modifications can be made applicable to all training schools.

Among other things it will be their duty to decide upon the necessary qualifications for applicants, the standards of examination, the term of probation and to provide for other emergencies. My object at present is to put before you the leading points; when these are settled the rest can, I think, be comparatively easily arranged.

The daily division of work for the eight-hour system could be made to work very nicely and interfere little, if any, with the present hours for meals by taking as a basis the hours 4 and 4 for some of the nurses, and 6 and 2 for the remainder. For instance, in a ward of thirty patients, with six nurses, supposing the entire staff comes on at 7 A. M. Two are sent off at 11 A. M. (1st dinner) 2; same to return from 7 until 11 P. M. (1st supper) 2. Four and four hours work.

Two off from 11 until 1 P. M. (1st dinner); with same two on from 1 until 5 P. M. (1st supper). Four and four hours work.

Two on from 7 until 1 P. M. (2d dinner); same two on from 5 until 7 P. M. (2d supper). Six and two hours work.

The night nurse from 11 P. M. until 7 A. M.

In this way either of the hours 7 A. M. until 11 P. M. may be taken, or hours from 6:30 A. M. to 10:30 P. M., or hours from 6 A. M. to 10 P. M. With this plan the nurses' classes and lectures could very well be arranged, and one, two or more nurses could be sent off at once, according to the condition of the wards. In this way the full staff could be on during the busy hours of the morning, and there would always be two nurses in the ward during meal-time. The hours of the head nurse and her first assistant, or senior, who would always be a third year nurse, should be so arranged that one or the other should be in the ward at all times during the day, and that both should never be absent at the same time.

These are some of the conditions under which I think the three years' course could be successfully adopted. It would possibly not be advisable to try to alter the present condition at one stroke, but to make the change gradually, so that in the course of the next five years the new system could be adopted in all of our good schools. Another consideration in connection with the subject is the co-operation of the larger with the smaller hospitals, but this I must leave to be discussed at some other time.

In conclusion, I would suggest that a chairman and commitee be appointed from the present convention to draw up a plan based somewhat upon the lines which have been suggested in this paper. That this plan, after having been duly considered, should be forwarded by the committee to the authorities of the various hospitals for their consideration and approval, and that the committee should ask that a trial of such a scheme may be permitted for a certain length of time in certain hospitals selected for that purpose in order that it may be thoroughly tested, after which some action may be taken, as the results of such trials would seem to indicate.

V

NURSING IN THE SMALLER HOSPITALS AND IN THOSE DEVOTED TO THE CARE OF SPECIAL FORMS OF DISEASE.

V

NURSING IN THE SMALLER HOSPITALS AND IN THOSE DEVOTED TO THE CARE OF SPECIAL FORMS OF DISEASE.*

I.—The various types of hospitals.
II.—Their methods of nursing.
III.—Five better methods suggested.
IV.—Plea for co-operative nursing.

I F I have to begin with an apology, and ask you not to criticise too sharply the crudeness of the paper which I shall present to you to-day, I cannot nevertheless accept the entire responsibility, for I feel that the fault lies also partly with circumstances and partly with our esteemed chairman. The subject was first assigned to Miss Palmer, but she found her time so occupied on assuming the duties of superintendent of the Rochester City Hospital that she wrote that it was impossible for her to prepare the paper. Our chairman in casting about for a substitute and knowing my good nature of old, has taken an unfair advantage of that knowledge. While I feel that she has conferred an honor by putting this

---

* Annual Convention American Superintendents' Society of Training Schools for Nurses, Baltimore, 1897.

task upon me, I am convinced that I have assumed a burden which is too heavy for me. The subject is one upon which I would speak gladly only after months of careful study; as it is too important and far-reaching to be touched upon lightly and in the short time at my disposal I have not been able to grapple with it with any great satisfaction to myself.

The question of providing nursing in the smaller hospitals and in those devoted to the care of special forms of disease is not a new one. I am sure that many of us in days gone by, as well as at the present time, have turned and are still turning the problem over and over in our minds. We have pondered it in the night season, and have had it with us as a continuous underlying current of thought through our busy working hours. For there is no doubt that this class of nursing goes far towards the making or un-undoing of our present system of caring for the sick both inside and outside of hospitals; its influence is far-reaching, and largely by the results obtained in these institutions will the profession of nursing rise or fall. It is, therefore, a problem that demands our most careful consideration and deliberation; it is not to be taken up lightly or passed over hastily, but discussed carefully and kept before us, until, as a convention, we are satisfied that the system of nursing in other than our large general hospitals has been made as perfect as possible.

We will first take a brief survey of this class of institutions and then consider their work and influence upon the nursing profession and their relation to the large hospitals.

In making up our list of hospitals we find that we have, indeed, a varied selection. There is the small general hospital, hospitals for children, for the general diseases of women, for women and children, for obstetrical cases, for gynæcological cases, and private hospitals for the insane. Again we have hydrotherapeutic establishments, special hospitals for the carrying out of the rest cure and for the treatment of nervous disorders, private hospitals and sanatoriums, hospitals in connection with large industrial enterprises, factories, railroads and mines ,emergency hospitals. hospitals for infectious and contagious diseases and those devoted to diseases of the eye, ear and throat. But, besides these hospitals, we have another large class of institutions which provides homes for the poor and feeble and which necessarily have wards connected with them. These are called by various names, such as homes and infirmaries, but inasmuch as part at least of their work is connected with the nursing of the sick, they are to be considered in this respect as hospitals.

Hospitals of one kind or another would then appear to be almost numerous enough. They form a network which reaches from ocean to ocean and from the north to the extreme south of the land. But it may be said that while the number of large hospitals hardly exceeds one hundred, the smaller are many times as numerous.

The existence of these small and special hospitals are the outcome of various factors. Some have been founded from pure philanthropy or as memorials of departed friends; others are the monuments of wealthy people, who wish to perpetuate their names, and in a country where fortunes are made as rapidly as in America this form of bequest is not unusual. Others, again, are integral parts of medical schools or universities, and their existence is demanded by the medical professors as necessary adjuncts to medical instruction. But, perhaps, a larger class still is the result of specialization among physicians, who open private hospitals, or so-called sanitariums, in which their own particular class of patients is cared for.

A study of the past and present history of hospitals, and more especially those of the last class, goes to show that the possibility of establishing and carrying on so many various hospitals and the continuous increase in their numbers is in a large measure due to the present system of nursing. Previous to the organization of Training Schools for Nurses, and for some years after, we find comparatively few hospitals in existence; but with the advent and suc-

cess of the trained nurse the question of providing for
the proper care of the sick in hospitals was solved,
and forthwith we find both physicians and laymen
rushing into hospital construction, with the result that
we have numbers of hospitals in operation to-day,
with much to be grateful for in connection with them
and not a few things to deplore.

Of those with which we are dealing at present, the
small general hospital probably ranks first in point
of usefulness, as it opens its doors at one time or another to all of the diseases for which the special hospitals are designed. Certainly, last in rank comes the
private hospital or sanitarium, opened by the specialist for his own particular patients and for his own
personal profit.

That any kind of a hospital which does its duty
by its patients has a perfect right to exist would seem
to be beyond question. Nevertheless it must be insisted that each owes a duty to the public as well
and must be open to commendation or censure, according to the system employed in providing proper
nursing for its sick. Upon investigation we find several methods employed. Some have organized training schools or offer a post-graduate course to nurses
from the smaller schools. Others, again, employ
graduate trained nurses. In a few co-operative nursing is established, one school undertaking the care
of two or more hospitals. Still others are under the

care of religious orders, and a few employ a corps of paid attendants who have never attended any regular school.

These various hospitals we may divide into three groups: (1) The small general hospital or cottage hospital, containing from fifty to seventy-five or one hundred beds. Hospitals for children, for women and children, lying-in hospitals, hospitals for gynæcological diseases, for nervous disorders and for rest cure cases.

(2) The very small general hospital, providing from six to forty beds. Sanitariums, hydrotherapeutic establishments, hospitals for infectious and contagious diseases, emergency hospitals, institutions for the insane, railroad and similar hospitals, and eye, ear and throat infirmaries.

(3) Infirmaries and homes. Hospitals for incurables.

With but few exceptions it will be found that the nursing in the first and second groups is done by training schools established in connection with each hospital. With many of the institutions in the third group we also find training schools; others, again, are cared for by paid attendants by the post-graduate system and by paid trained nurses.

But, unfortunately, in all of the groups, dozens or even hundreds of hospitals are met with containing only from six to ten or twenty beds, and yet main-

taining training schools for nurses. The well-known
circular of information is sent out offering apparently the same advantages as the larger schools. The
course of instruction covers two years; the pupils
must be of a certain age, though frequently they are
taken as young as eighteen; they have certain hours
on duty, time for rest and recreation. It would appear also they have the same classes and lectures, for,
according to the prospectus, they are instructed "in
the general care of the sick, making beds, changing
bed and body linen, giving baths, dressing bed sores,
making bandages, in the application of fomentations
and of poultices, in cupping, leeching" and other ac-
complishments. We meet again and again the same
old list, but whether it means much or little, or less
than nothing, it is often impossible to say. Certainly
for the uninitiated and ignorant woman who knows
nothing of hospitals it is a fine bait. But as an addition we have the statement that after the probation
month the pupil will receive each month for the first
year a certain number of dollars and an increased
number of dollars monthly for the second year, and
this ostensibly to cover the cost of uniform and text
books. Finally examinations are held and certificates of qualification are presented. But when one
reads in the "Trained Nurse" such statements as
this, "Two nurses graduated from the ———— hos-

pital with all honors,'' one certainly is justified in inferring that honors were easy in such cases.

Now why is it that all these small and special hospitals adopt this method of nursing, and offer such inducements, and why is it that the demand is supplied by so many women? In the first place competition is so great in these days that the public demands, and rightly so, to be well taken care of. Again, physicians know that with trained nursing their results will be better and will not lend their names or allow themselves to be connected with any institution that is apparently lacking in this respect. A third and most potent reason is the fact that training schools are cheaper and the pupils are easier to manage than graduate nurses. In fact, in many instances the pupils are a source of distinct profit, for in some of these schools they are required not only to do the hospital nursing, but are also sent out to private duty, sometimes for weeks at a time, during their two years' service, while the $10 or $15 per week which they earn goes towards the support of the hospital and school, and in some instances forms quite a large item. This is perfectly well known, despite the fact that one never reads of the nurses as financial benefactors, all the glory and honor of that kind going to the managing body of the institution.

Perhaps the best excuse which could be urged in defense of the system is that more and better work and a stricter discipline are possible in a training school than can be obtained where graduate trained nurses or attendants are employed.

Again, the apparently liberal offer of an education and compensation at the same time attracts women, good, bad and indifferent, in sufficiently large numbers to keep the vacancies filled, if one is not over particular as to requirements. And perhaps it is too much to expect that a woman who has never seen the inside of a hospital should be competent to differentiate between the different grades of schools and their advantages. The compensation is also an added inducement, and she may not realize that for a present small gain she is sacrificing future higher professional standing and better opportunities. I must add also that people have not yet quite got over the habit of thinking that if a woman is a failure at everything else she is at least fit to go into a hospital and become a nurse, and unfortunately it happens that, although such an incompetent has no possible chance for entrance into the general hospital school, she is still received with open arms into the private and special hospitals.

The small general hospital, with fifty beds or more, is generally justified in having attached to it an organized training school. The so-called cottage hospitals found in the smaller cities or in thickly populated country districts have a comparatively wide

scope. They meet a need which can be supplied in
no other way, and their usefulness is at once apparent. One occasionally reads, in the nursing magazines, short articles in favor of the training afforded
by these cottage hospitals as compared with that
obtainable in a large general hospital in the city.
It is argued that the nurse is better equipped for
her work in that she comes into more direct contact
with her superintendent and the physicians, and also because from the very smallness of the field she
is able to study and become well acquainted with
any case that is of peculiar importance. But certainly it would appear that if a large general training school is properly systematized and managed, it
must naturally follow that the pupil gets all and
a great deal more than she can in a small hospital.
Where this is not the case there is something wrong
with the management of the larger school. As a
proof that pupils from the smaller hospitals do not
always find their training sufficient, superintendents
of the larger general schools could tell how often application is made to them by graduates from these,
as well as from schools belonging to special hospitals,
stating that they wish for a larger and more varied
experience. We know, however, that many of our
small general training schools do excellent work and
turn out competent graduates. Where they are offi-
cered by graduates from   large   general   **training**

schools, who are good managers and disciplinarians, and are enthusiastic in their work, every opportunity is seized and utilized for the advantage of the pupils, who can thus secure a thorough and fairly wide training. Again, when the nurse has graduated she often finds her field of work right in the town or surrounding country where she is among friends.

The amount of good accomplished by these cottage hospitals, both within and without their walls, is inestimable. They fill a long felt want and rob illness in town and country of half its terrors, and are of unspeakable comfort to the physicians, who are usually their promoters and warm suporters.

In some instances, particularly in hospitals connected with churches, we find the nursing done by members of religious orders, sisters or deaconesses. For some reasons it seems to me to be regretted that in some church hospitals the sisters are giving up this branch of their work in favor of nurses and are establishing training schools in connection with these institutions. Might it not possibly be better that a certain per cent. of the sisters should be regularly instructed in nursing, so that from their number a permanent staff of skilled workers would always be obtainable?

Turning to the remainder of the first group, which are all established for the care of some particular class of patients, we find, alas, that training schools

again abound, and the same attractive circulars are
being issued for the enlightenment of applicants.
With few exceptions, these hospitals are established
in cities and therefore cannot plead isolation. No
doubt women who enter these schools become well
grounded in the care of one particular class of patients and their diseases, but it is absurd to claim
that she graduates from there with a thorough, all-
round training in both the practice and theory of her
work, which would justify her in assuming the title
of trained nurse. It is true that she may make the
care of that particular disease her specialty and attempt nothing else, but even then, everything else
being equal, she cannot long be as efficient even in
this limited sphere as the graduate from the general
hospital, who, aided by an intelligent and varied
knowledge, supplemented by wide experience and
practice, can speedily adapt herself to any particular
class of cases. If we think of the future of the women who enter these hospitals, it would seem that but
little can be said in justification of the managers of
such hospitals in their position as organizers of training schools. We are compelled to think that the welfare of their pupil nurses with them is a matter of
no importance. To have the patients well cared for
with as little expense and friction and with as much
ease as possible is their first consideration. Experience may have shown that this end can be most easily

attained by establishing a training school, but we may well ask whether the means are justifiable. It is puerile to argue that the pupil nurse is a free agent and need not enter such a school or stay after she is there. But can we reasonably expect that a woman who is ignorant of hospitals and their methods can be in a position to differentiate between what is advisable or inadvisable, more especially when the institution has the support of many good names?

I do not mean that these special hospitals do not turn out some excellent nurses. I believe quite to the contrary, for there are always some women bright and clever enough to profit by their work no matter where they are placed; the greater the pity that their privileges are not broader and more complete. Many of these special hospitals undoubtedly fill distinct needs and it may be to the interest of both patients and science to have them in our midst. Children's hospitals, private hospitals for the carrying out of the rest cure and the treatment of nervous patients and separate hospitals for the insane are necessities. It does not, however, follow that they should each organize a training school. That hospitals and sanitariums opened by individuals for their own private gain should have in connection with them training schools for nurses, is a condition worthy of the severest condemnation.

One especially glaring instance has just come under my notice. I have recently been told of a private special hospital owned by one man which accommodates thirty patients; his training school for nurses numbers twenty pupils. The promoter's sole plea is that he tried graduate nurses but they did so badly that he was obliged to open a school. These same graduates were no doubt products of institutions equally as bad as his own.

Such examples are repeated over and over again and yet graduates from such schools receive the same title and claim from the public and their fellows the same recognition awarded to trained nurses, who have given of their best time and strength to qualify themselves in well equipped schools to do their work thoroughly and be an honor to their profession. Every year these hospitals and graduates are on the increase until they threaten to take entire possesion of the land. Right-minded, deep-thinking men and women among the laity who interest themselves in hospital work are averse to this system of multiplying small half-equipped training schools, and the question has been put to me, and I am sure to other superintendents many times, What other way is there? What else can be suggested which would seem to promote better results than those obtained by the methods now generally in vogue?

Exclusive of training schools we have five courses left open to us. The nursing could be undertaken

(1) by the graduates of smaller schools willing to give their services in return for a post-graduate course under competent instructors, (2) By paid competent graduate nurses, (3) By attendants under the supervision of trained nurses, (4) By adopting the system of co-operative nursing, (5) By members of religious orders, previously trained for these duties.

Of these various methods I would here, as in my paper on ''Educational Standards for Nurses,'' make my special plea for co-operative nursing whenever such a scheme is feasible. This method I am happy to say has already been put into practice in some few schools. For nine years the Illinois Training School, of Chicago, has successfully provided for the nursing of two large institutions with its pupils, thereby adding largely to the experience and competency of the pupils and at the same time helping to elevate the standard of nursing work. It has also been for some years in operation in Milwaukee, and in 1894 we read that ''a new system has been introduced into the Utica, N. Y., Hospital, whereby pupils from the Faxton Hospital Training School do the nursing.'' The writer adds, ''The cost to the city is less than formerly even should twice the number of nurses be on duty there.'' The Emergency Hospital, of San Francisco, is provided for by pupils of the Children's Hospital; of the Sloan Maternity, New York, by pupils from the New York Training School. In Washington the Columbia and Children's Hospital arranged to interchange pupils, and at one time there was a suggestion that the Garfield should unite with them. Certainly if such special hospitals, as those for children, women and children, lying-in hospitals, and hospitals for gynæcological and for nervous cases are so situated in the cities that they could co-operate with a general hospital or other institutions, they owe it to the women they take into their schools to do so. The first move must naturally come from the trustees or boards of management, but the actual success depends wholly upon the superintendents of the various schools, and now that we are getting on a more common plane as to teaching and requirements for entrance and graduation, the plan seems more feasible than before. But its accomplishment will require much patience and self-sacrifice on the part of some of our number and the only certain reward which I can offer to them is the feeling that they will have rendered possible the attainment of the greater good to the greater number.

Some special hospitals offer a post-graduate course to graduates from other schools who wish for further training. The weak point in this system lies in the fact that they canot offer an all-round experience, and if a graduate from one special hospital enters another of a similar kind offering her a post-graduate course, she only adds to her experience the knowledge of one other special disease. Only when a woman has already a general training and then enters a post-graduate school for the sake of perfecting herself in the cure of one particular class of cases is the post-graduate course made use of in the right way; unless, as already suggested by Miss Davis in her paper on "A Post-Graduate Course," we can find some general hospital whose managers will be willing to organize its school on the post-graduate basis and thus offer opportunities for further development to all kinds of graduates.

Training schools in connection with hospitals for the insane are as yet few in number, but the tendency to increase them is growing and undoubtedly in the care of this class of patients there is room for much improvement. But can these hospitals any more than any special hospitals offer sufficient variety in nursing to produce all-round trained nurses? Experience shows that their graduates also try for admittance into general training schools and are willing to give two more years of their time without pay in order to gain more experience in their work. It would seem that the plan adopted by the superintendent of one hospital for the insane might be a good one, that is to appoint a certain number of trained nurses as supervisors and let their staff of assistants be paid permanent attendants. Such also might be the system in emergency hospitals, infirmaries and homes and hydrotherapeutic establishments. Hospitals for infectious diseases, the eye, ear and throat infirmaries should certainly be under the care of graduate trained nurses or else under the co-operative system.

Such plans as I have outlined are given to you in the way of suggestions. Some of them have been tried successfully. No doubt there remain others, still better, to be discovered. In any case it is a duty incumbent upon each trained nurse to use her efforts against the establishment of any more small half equipped schools and to use her efforts towards improving, where it is possible, those already in existence, and the strong distinction between thoroughly equipped schools and the half-equipped ones should be to put the best schools on a purely educational basis, withdraw the monthly allowance, increase the time of training, and in return offer a broad and liberal education to women who would become trained nurses.

The writer would beg in conclusion that any one who may read this paper will remember that it has been written entirely without prejudice or without any feeling of ''looking down'' upon the small or special schools. It is simply a plea for the broader and more liberal education of all who call themselves trained nurses. It is only meant as an effort to draw

us as a profession nearer together, to place nursing
the continent over on a distinct and sure basis beyond all questioning. It has been said that "the
country is swarming with ill-paid stenographers who
cannot spell or punctuate, with starving sewing-wo-
men who sew badly, with cooks who do not know how
to cook, and in many cases with so-called trained
nurses who are lacking in tact, good manners, and
education." Some women are given the popular term
"born nurses" when they are especially remarkable
for good sense and adaptability; but we know that
nurses are *made* not born, and the rule has but few
exceptions, that it is the woman whose general education is the best who is able to do one particular
thing best. If this be true in the simplest things,
how much more is training required for work as
complicated as nursing. Dr. Weir Mitchell says that
a woman to be a nurse requires education, tact, good
sense, good manners, and good health. Given all
these requirements, and nothing less should be the
standard, we owe it to such a woman in preparing
her to be a trained nurse to give her the best that
the work of nursing affords. By making this our
standard, by lengthening the term of service and
lessening the daily practical work, so that her brain
may be in a good condition to understand the theory
of nursing, and she may do her practical work with

more understanding, and by bringing these small and special hospitals into line and touch with our large general schools we shall all be the gainers.

MODERN HOSPITAL NURSING.

MODERN HOSPITAL NURSING.*

IT WAS in a military hospital amid the tumult of battle in the great Crimean war that the modern system of nursing found its birthplace. Here came into existence a force born to do battle forevermore in the never ceasing struggle for life. As the child of that war has increased in years it has grown mightily in strength until to-day although still young, its power is recognized in the East and West, the North and South. There is hardly a mission in foreign lands that has not its skilled nurses. In plague-stricken India, in the wars of both East and West; in the South with its fatal fever, and in the lands of the North, wheresoever plague, pestilence or famine are to be found, there too side by side is the trained nurse, quietly, silently doing battle. Even in our every-day lives we can scarcely turn our eyes in any direction without encountering her. There is not a modern hospital of which she is not an integral part. Scientific medicine would find it hard to do without her. In infirmaries, asylums, day nurseries, schools, church parishes, in the solitary sick-room, and among the poor in their homes she is doing her

---

* Opening of New Lakeside Hospital, Cleveland, 1898.

work. To few is it given as to Florence Nightingale, the heroine of the Crimea and the patron Saint of Nurses to see so great results in so brief a time from the seed she has sown. And it is the light of her lamp at night that still throws its shadow on the wall of many a hospital ward the world over, for none among her followers have a clearer or more penetrating insight into things pertaining to hospitals and nursing than has Miss Nightingale to-day. Long may that light with its inspiring flame burn among us.

Something over eight years ago in connection with the opening of that hospital which is the heart and centre of scientific medicine in America and in the possession of which medical men the continent over feel a truly pardonable pride, it was my privilege to speak briefly of the aims and objects of training schools for nurses. These eight years have seen many changes in the thought, work and methods of the medical profession—changes which have necessarily exercised a great influence upon the training of nurses.

At the present time it would be considered out of date and only a sign of ignorance for a physician to affirm that all he requires of a nurse is that she should be a well working automaton to carry out his orders, and that he would prefer that she should not know even part of his reasons for what is done for the patient. Such an idea, popular as it once was, has now fortunately become antiquated. The progress of medicine itself has taught that a very different intelligence is required of a nurse. The science of bacteriology which in a few years has conclusively demonstrated the causes of many diseases and her sister "preventive medicine" require one and all who meddle with medicine whether as physicians or nurses to be people of intelligence. So long as drugs were looked upon as "cure-alls" for all bodily ailments, an automaton who would administer the doses at certain intervals may have perhaps answered every purpose; but at present some of our remedial or preventive measures would seem to the uninitiated to appear too vague and even far-fetched so that it would be impossible to insure a conscientious carrying out of them unless the intelligence were appealed to. What for instance are we to understand by cleanliness? For the uninitiated the sense is very clear. And yet there is a deeper meaning which can only be appreciated by those who have mastered at least the broad principles of bacteriology. How hopeless and dull, not to say irritating, would be the many washings and the various aseptic precautions which are now required from the nurse by the physician unless she had learned from bacteriology to appreciate the fact that there exists a surgical, a microscopical cleanliness. For this purpose then the nurse must have some knowledge of the broad principles of bacteriology To fully appreciate the effect upon the patient of the air he breathes and the food he eats she must know something of ventilation and hygiene. For the proper care of the body she has to go to physiology. To become acquainted with the best forms and preparations of food by which the greatest possible amount of bodily resistance to disease are established and maintained she must profit by the demonstrations given in the diet school. Such matters of detail are usually entrusted to the nurse. She alone can devote to them such constant and unremitting attention as are necessary. It is true that the physician can lay down a broad, general outline of such matters, but the details—the little things that matter so much—must of necessity be often left to the nurse, and how shall she supply all this without intelligence and a proper education in her profession. How can she profit by this special education unless she brings to it a mind already trained to think and comprehend, a groundwork to build upon. In hospitals the doctors may be temporarily off duty, the nurse is always in charge. Her candle goeth not out by night and it is to her watchfulness and intelligent care that the patients are in the main committed through the night. She must be taught how much and how little she can do and when it is necessary to call in further aid.

But the training of a nurse in a hospital does not

deal merely with book-learning or with clinical methods. It carries with it the building up of character. The nurse is taught that the most scrupulous honesty is necessary in all her work, that any omission, whether it come about wilfully or through ignorance, may be productive of the most serious results; that one step in aseptic technique omitted or slurred over may be paid for by the life of the patient committed to her charge. May we not then regard the training school of a modern hospital as a place not only for preparing women to undertake properly the care of the sick, but also where properly selected women are given such moral and educational advantages that they may go forth equipped to aid in the practical solution of some of the various social problems which can be solved only by help of intelligent womanly work?

She is limited only by her own limitations, for as she shows her ability to fill them, other fields of usefulness are being opened up to her. A further progress or evolution from hospital, private nursing and district nursing dates from four years ago when two trained nurses in New York City formed a Nurses' Settlement in one of the most densely populated tenement districts. From rooms in a tenement house the headquarters have been removed to a good sized private dwelling in which eight nurses now make their home. At present there are three such settlements in New York, which do an infinite variety of work besides attending upon the sick. The members of these settlements have become a power for good among much misery. Their opportunities for the acquirement of practical knowledge concerning the problems connected with the poor in all great cities has lately been recognized by the election of one of their number as a member of the Sanitary Health Association of New York City, while in London a trained nurse has just been appointed on the London School Board. In the same city a nurse is regularly employed by the Corporation to teach practical hygiene in the poor districts.

Another movement of interest is that which aims at the introduction of trained nurses in families of only moderate means. In some cities, associations have been formed to provide a nurse who attends for one or more hours a day for a moderate fee and who sees that such arrangements are made that the patient is taken proper care of.

Thus it will be seen that in many ways the profession is broadening out and the graduate members are practically taking their part in aiding in the propagation and advancement of preventive medicine.

Within the profession itself also we are not standing still, but are ever aiming at improvements upon older methods. We have now an organized association of superintendents of training schools who, at the expenditure of not a little time, energy and money, are doing much to bring about some degree of uniformity among the different schools. Their aim is to establish, as far as possible, uniform standards as regards requirements for entrance, the curriculum, and the granting of certificates. The best schools are beginning to increase the time of training from two to three years, and are thus improving the quality of the graduate nurse. If they have lessened the quantity by these means, they have done no harm. This distinct effort to put training schools upon a higher educational basis has also been furthered by those schools, who have, at the same time, introduced the non-payment system, and who, while asking the nurse to forego a present remuneration, havè guaranteed to her in return for her work a thorough education, as well as practical training. Under these circumstances, it was only just that more time for study, lectures and demonstrations should be given to the pupil nurse, and that all her energies should not be exhausted in the routine work of the wards, which should now occupy her only for eight hours out of twenty-four. While some schools have extended their course to three years, and others have adopted the non-payment system, it is to be regreted that at present in only one or two hospitals have the hours of daily practical work been reduced to eight, the average time required still being usually from 10 to 11 hours.

As a nurse who has watched all these changes with keen interest, I take peculiar pleasure in assisting at the opening of the Lakeside Hospital because it is the first hospital on record supported by private contributions that opens its school for nurses upon a purely educational basis. The women are to be congratulated who enter this training school as pupil nurses. The fact that the trustees of the hospital in its construction and sanitary arrangements have given every thought for the care and the well-being of the patients augurs well for the fulfillment of the obligations which they have taken upon themselves in accepting pupils in their training school. Honor and credit are due to their broad-minded and far-seeing policy which insists that patients can be properly taken care of only by intelligent and well-trained nurses. This school offers to its pupils a three years course of instruction with eight hours practical work in the wards. The pupils receive no payment but are furnished a thorough systematic practical and theoretical education in return for their work. As a result the women who enter as pupils will be those who come seeking knowledge and who have high ideals. The commercially minded woman who looks only to the dollars and cents can have no place here. Fortunate indeed are those whose privilege it is to study nursing at this time and to become a part of the working force of such a hospital. Of friends she finds plenty, of enemies few. She can not be classed with the "new woman," for her art is ancient history and extends through the ages. We read of fair ladyes nursing their stricken knights, of Elaine tending the wounded Launcellot, or of the Good Samaritan binding up wounds, pouring in oil and wine. Nor do we lack the Master's reply to the question, "When saw we thee sick or in prison, and ministered unto thee?" "Even as ye did it unto the least of one of these my brethren." The woman in this profession needs no pity bestowed upon her; her days are all rounded out in absorbing work and interest and so are happy ones. It is exceedingly interesting to visit old St. Bartholomew's hospital in London. Over 500 years have passed since its doors were first opened to the sick. Its history is most impressive, and as one follows it step by step through its buildings one realizes as never before that such a hospital is not only for to-day and to-morrow or for our own short lives, but that its life and influence will extend far into the future and will bear with it the lives of its men and women bound up with it.

To the building up a fabric of personal education and personal character; to the preparation for boundless opportunities for good work in the world, to happy useful lives, and to the welfare of future generations are the women dedicated who become part of this new Hospital and Training School, the inception of which we are here to witness. As an older member in this profession of nursing I rejoice in its high standing and the opportunities offered to its nurses, and as the representative of the Associated Trained Nurses in the United States and Canada I bid it welcome and God-speed.

VII

THE AIMS, METHODS AND SPIRIT
OF THE ASSOCIATED ALUMNÆ
OF TRAINED NURSES OF
THE UNITED STATES.

THE AIMS, METHODS AND SPIRIT OF THE ASSOCIATED ALUMNAE OF TRAINED NURSES OF THE UNITED STATES.*

O N one other occasion it has been my privilege to make the opening address at a gathering of trained nurses, and in the fact that in that first meeting was laid the foundation stone for this present organization lies the exceedingly great pleasure I now take in announcing the opening of the first annual meeting of the Nurses' Associated Alumnæ of the United States and Canada. The occasions have a certain similarity, in that the former had the distinction of being the first occasion in the history of trained nursing in America on which nurses had met together to discuss affairs dealing with the various interests of their profession, while this second meeting heralds the beginning of organized work among nurses. But, from another point of view, the two meetings show a marked dissimilarity. The first presented an unorganized body of women with indefinite views and an uncertain future. To the present one we come as an

---

* First Annual Convention of the Associated Alumnae of Trained Nurses, New York, 1898.

organized, representative body with definite objects and ready to deal with some of the problems which, with the growth of the profession, have presented themselves for solution. Among the papers read and discussed at the Congress of Nurses in 1893 were two that had a direct bearing upon this present association. One, by Miss Edith Draper, was on ''The Benefits of Alumnæ Associations;'' the other, by Miss McIsaac, on ''The Necessity of an American Nurses' Association.'' These two papers ably outlined the necessity for development in nursing work along the lines of organization. Under the stimulus of these papers, as well as that which was naturally evoked by the meeting together in a common interest, the hitherto unexpressed thought or feeling on the part of different superintendents that more co-operation and community of ideas in the general work would be helpful and a necessity, found vent, with the result that the American Society of Superintendents of Nurses was organized. This was the most vital and only really important result of that first meeting. The avowed objects of the Superintendents' Society are ''To further the best interests of the nursing profession by establishing a universal standard of training and by promoting fellowship among its members by meetings, papers and discussions and by interchange of opinions.'' From the beginning it was very clear to the society that the broader outlook for nurses must first come through organized school alumnæ associations of the graduates before anything could be done toward establishing a national association on anything like a permanent basis. It also recognized the advantage to the busy graduate nurses of having a body already organized to relieve them of the burden and responsibility of all the various details involved in the formation of an organization. And, appreciating this fact, what more natural than that these superintendents should declare themselves willing to undertake this work looking toward the higher and better interests of the nursing profession and of the graduates, many of whom these superintendents were responsible for making trained nurses. Papers and discussions were therefore prepared on "Training School Alumnæ Associations" for each of the first two annual meetings. The second of these papers, by Miss Palmer, read February, 1895, with the purpose of showing the available material for a national association, gave a report of the number of alumnæ associations in existence at that date. From a list of 164 training schools there were thirty-one organized alumnæ associations or clubs; eighteen reported no organization, and fifty-five were not heard from. No attempt had been made, however, to classify these bodies with reference to their eligibility for membership in a national association. At the time of the meeting in Chicago there were possibly half a dozen alumnæ associations organized. The fact that thirty-one were already in existence after the lapse of only two years was a gratifying evidence of the mind of the nurses on the subject.

At the third annual meeting of the Superintendents' Society a very comprehensive paper was read by Miss L. L. Dock on "A National Association for Nurses and Its Legal Organization." After the discussion that followed, it was moved that a committee of five be appointed by the Chair, to select seven others, who should form the nucleus of a convention to prepare a national constitution, and that they should secure an equal number of delegates from among the oldest alumnæ societies, who should not be holding hospital positions, to unite with them in drawing up a constitution. This motion was carried, and it was also ordered that a report should be made at the next annual meeting. In accordance with this resolution the committee submitted its first, which was also its final report, at the annual meeting held in Baltimore in February, 1897, as follows:—

"Your committee reports that, immediately after the last annual session of this society, your committee met to consider methods of forming a convention for the work of organizing a national association. Other members of this society who were invited to join with them were Miss Nutting, Miss Draper, Miss Snively, Miss Maxwell, Miss Hutchinson, Mrs. Robb, Miss Palmer. Twelve representative alumnæ associations were chosen and were invited each to send one delegate to the convention. These alumnæ associations were the Massachusetts General, the Presbyterian (New York), Bellevue, the New York, the New Haven, the Orange Memorial, the Johns Hopkins, the University of Pennsylvania, the Philadelphia, the Brooklyn City, the Illinois and the Farrand. All accepted, and the first meeting of the convention took place at Manhattan Beach, on September 2, 1896. A constitution and by-laws were drafted for an association covering the United States and Canada, and a second meeting was appointed for February, 1897, in Baltimore, and at the same date as the meeting of this society. At this second meeting it is expected that the constitution will be adopted and officers elected.

"The expenses involved up to the time of the first meeting of the convention were met by this society; after that time by the alumnæ associations represented. "Respectfully submitted,

> "L. L. DOCK,
> "ISABEL M'ISAAC,
> "ISABEL MERRITT,
> "M. B. BROWN,
> "LUCY L. WALKER."

The result of the second meeting in Baltimore we have heard from the Secretary.

Such in brief is the history of the beginnings of this national organization of alumnæ associations of training schools. With the presentation of the report above also ends the responsibility of the Superintendents' Society, as a society, toward this organization, a responsibility so generously assumed by women, already crowded with work, in the best interests of the nursing profession in general and with absolutely no personal motives in view other than the good that may come to them individually as members of their several alumnæ societies. As one of their own members said in the discussion following Miss Dock's paper, ''Superintendents will form a very small part of this organization; it will be an association of independent women, who hope by organization to work many reforms.'' Just here at this parting of the ways, as it were, of the two societies, it would seem fitting in accepting this work at their hands and before entering upon a consideration of the affairs of the National Association, that we pause and move a vote of appreciation and thanks to the American Society of Superintendents of Nurses for their services of time, money and labor so freely expended in the higher interests of trained nurses and the nursing profession.

It seems like a brief dream as to time since that June of 1895, but a dreaming true as to results. So splendid have these results been thus far that I look forward into the future of the associated alumnæ with joy and with certainty that it will achieve greater and better things by nurses and for nurses than have ever yet come to pass. And with such a feeling and in such a spirit do I invite you to a consideration of the work before us at this meeting and of the future aims of the association.

This meeting is full of importance. We have first to consider our methods of work, arrangements of committees and constitutional amendments. The question of admitting the smaller schools into constitutional membership and with what limitations, is the most important one now before us. Recognizing the immense importance of very full discussions, it has been thought best that only one paper should be read at each session. These papers will deal with subjects that are of ethical and practical importance to us in beginning our work. We have one on ''The Duty and Opportunity of the Alumnæ.'' Another on ''The Best Means of Co-ordinating the Work of the General Association and Its Branches,'' which will deal with State and local organizations. A third will deal with finance and investment, and I trust will help to lay a foundation toward a future practical method of encouraging our members in thrift and economy. Feeling sure, then, that all our discussions will be characterized by a dignified, wisely conservative and generous spirit, I will now very briefly direct your attention to some of the problems and possibilities that the future holds for us and which should furnish us with inspiration and encouragement to be loyal and true to the trust that is committed to each individual member of this association.

The objects as outlined in our constitution may seem simple and few in the reading; and yet concealed in each there lies folded up the seed of many a plan and purpose that can only come to maturity in the fulness of time, when the work shall be lifted from our hands, as we become incapacitated, and carried on to loftier ideals and higher aims by the strong young hands, hearts and brains of future nurses. And remembering this, it may be as well if we begin by making haste slowly, but steadily and surely. For if we proceed on these lines from the first, we shall have less to regret and less to pull down later and shall end by accomplishing some little of real worth.

Our work for the first few years must, in the nature of things, be constructive. A code of ethics is the first object mentioned in the constitution. But it cannot be among the first to be realized, for such a code should be the central point of thought of the association, reaching out in its influence and inspiration to our most remote branches and toward which each individual member may look vibrant with a sense of personal responsibility toward the association and toward the highest standard attainable by nurses. It should stand for deeds and actions, not words and form. Were we, therefore, to appoint a committee to forthwith formulate a code of ethics, we should get words, but not the spirit. Surely, it will be better to wait until we have taken sufficient and better form in the matter of numbers and closer organization, to learn the mind of the greater number on what shall constitute our national code of ethics. But I would like to say, in passing, that it should be founded, not on the lines of that of any existing association or society, but should be formulated to meet our own special needs in our own particular way.

The second clause reads, "To elevate the standard of nursing education." If ethics is our central thought, here indeed is our central problem, embodying, as it will in its solution, the combined and unremitting interest and efforts of every single member. Its breadth and height and depth are of such dimensions that it will require the most earnest thought of various minds before we can begin to see our way clear to the necessary steps to take for its ultimate solution. Time will only permit me to suggest some of the lines upon which a working basis may possibly be found for the present.

We do not need more training schools, but better ones. We should aim to build up and strengthen those training schools that already exist and to discourage the establishment of others with insufficient means and unscholarly ideas. The organization of schools in the very small and specialty hospitals already appeal directly to us. We should work out some method by which the nursing in such hospitals could be undertaken whenever possible by the association. I believe the day will come when we shall see our way clear toward caring for many of this class of hospitals through its members. We should have no desire to prevent the organization of these small hospitals—we would not if we could, for they have their own particular place and mission to fill in the smaller places and for the specialties they stand for —but we must bear in mind that our first reason for being nurses is to tend, support and care for the helpless in the most efficient way possible. And if we can, as an organization, aid the trustees of hospitals in carrying out their responsibility of giving their patients the best of care by competent nurses, it is our distinct duty to do so, and to furnish them with a high grade of nursing at no greater cost than would be entailed by a small training school and untrained pupils, of which they would otherwise probably avail themselves. This system at the same time would help to materially lessen the number of inadequately trained nurses and, so far as instruction goes, would make the qualifications for membership in State or National associations practically the same for all trained nurses. It would also throw better material, and more of it, into the hands of the better equipped schools, and in this way increase the educational standard of our schools and raise the standard of requirements for women who wish to become trained nurses. Again, it would insure more continuous and agreeable work for a greater number of competent women, who prefer hospital work to other branches of nursing. Such a plan as this, however, can only be rendered feasible by having a supply of specially trained women ready to undertake these positions as superintendents in such hospitals, and by having funds in our treasury for the purpose of supplementing, where necessary, the salaries of the nurses. For we should not be willing to have nurses undertake institutional work for inadequate compensation. For this reason, therefore, it might be advisable, in the case of very poor hospitals, for the association to allow their members to undertake the nursing and at the same time to guarantee to them a fair and just remuneration in proportion to the degree of work and responsibility assumed. To insure proper nursing, then, in the poorer and smaller hospitals should be one of our purposes in having money and accepting bequests.

The organization of State and local branches is advisable as a factor in educational advancement. Their importance is manifest in many, but more especially in two ways:—First, because through them only can details of the work outlined by the main organization be successfully carried into effect; and, secondly, because from an educational standpoint the local alumnæ societies are of particular value, in that through them the educational interests of the individual graduate can be best fostered and properly cared for. As we all know, a hospital training does not represent the sum total of professional knowledge, and the successful nurse will be she who keeps abreast of the times. The opportunities for further study for the graduate beyond the regular undergraduate courses are often very limited, but where the different alumnæ associations of a city or locality become united, they can devise practical ways and means for the encouragement of systematic postgraduate study. It is a source of pleasure to note that in Brooklyn the alumnæ associations have already united their forces and are doing good work together.

But it is hardly less important that these local associations should have some outside interests as well. They should identify themselves with educational and philanthropic efforts and take part, so far as they can, outside in such movements, even when not strictly in their own line of work. In this way only will it be possible to avoid the danger of an association becoming narrow and selfish in its life. It is impossible to more than touch upon the educational side of these local associations. Their work will be hard, no doubt, and sometimes discouraging, but, on the other hand, they will have the enjoyment and benefit that comes from unity of purpose, from the element of variety that comes with the broader contact with others in the same work, from the free interchange of all the newest and best ideas outside of their own particular school, and from the added feeling of loyalty to their own society that such contact engenders. They should also lend their aid in endeavoring to direct philanthropy into the most effective channels. From the nature of their knowledge of sanitation and the laws of health, they should in the future have representation on educational boards, State Boards of Health, hospital and training school boards. They may thus use their influence in forming a correct public sentiment in matters of social reform. Another sphere of activity in which associations may engage is the opening of new avenues of branches of work affording means for employment outside of the usual ones of hospital or private nursing. The plan for visiting nurses has already been successfully inaugurated, and at the present time a local society in New York is endeavoring to redeem the application of mechanicotherapeutics from the hands of charlatans and place it in the hands of trained nurses, where it belongs. Last, but not least, there is the nurses' settlement work. In all such ways and many more may the influence of the association be unbounded, not only upon those who directly share its privileges, but upon the community at large. And so we may gradually grow into the third object of our association—that of being useful and honored.

And now just a word on the subject of finances. It would not seem out of place for an association of this kind to interest itself in the future financial welfare of its members. For present needs, in case of illness, members of their own school alumnæ associations are assured through sick benefit funds, but it is for the years to come that provision should be made, and that through the thrift of the nurse herself. It is a well known fact that nurses are not very provident as a class, but could some plan be evolved by which systematic saving would be stimulated it would result in a feeling of security and independence for the nurse as to her future maintenance.

It seems to me that there is one feature of work which should prove of the utmost value and aid in helping us to make known and carry out the various objects which have been referred to—I mean the development of publications and of literature dealing with matters which concern directly or indirectly our profession. Just on what basis these developments may be best advanced I will leave for the present. Suffice it to say that this is a point which will bear much discussion and thought, and about which any ultimate plan can only be the result of a consensus of opinions.

Thus brifly have we passed in review some of the objects that we have to work for. Many nurses have asked and more will ask, "What is there in it for me if I join the alumnæ association?" In answer we would say through the alumnæ association of your school and the national associations all the possibilities that we have pointed out will be opened to you. But more remains; through them you will gain the broader and more unselfish life that comes to each woman who has ideals in her work an does not regard it merely from a commercial standpoint. The first president of Wellesley College said to the college students, "You do not go to college to earn your bread —not this only—but to make every mouthful of bread more nourishing sweeter. It is to learn how to live —to make life, not a living. You may forget some of your Greek and Latin verbs, your geometry, history, but you need not forget your ideals. They may be yours always, or, better than this, they may be realized, for the students of to-day must be a great body marching toward the solution of problems we have not yet solved. In you we may have our meanings of the stars." How aptly may this be applied to trained nurses of to-day, into whose hands the pioneer nurses in America now place this nursing work, to be carried on to a higher plane to which the eyes of the world may look up, not down, learning to work together in a common interest, with harmony,

method, and in a spirit of self-sacrifice strengthen-
ing the intelligent loyalty and efficient service of
each member for her own alumnæ association. It
is very natural to look at the outset for the difficulties ahead, but I can foresee few that may not be
overcome if skillfuly attacked. Necessarily, there
is a great amount of labor involved, and patience
will be necessary before we can hope to realize any
definite results. What we need is to quietly and
steadily persevere. Our methods should be direct,
simple and easy to understand for any one, and the
spirit that underlies them should be generous and
impersonal and tempered by a wise conservatism.

Finally, the interests of the individual should be
one with those of the whole association. It is impossible to make too strong an appeal to your *esprit
de corps.* Each member should see that the association and its work is loyally sustained in the years
that are to come. Such work, though it may be well
organized, will always need this individual attention
and feeling of personal responsibilty from the members, if we would look toward the day when the ideal
nurse will be the rule and not the exception; her influence felt in the home, the hospital, our educational
institutions and over the broad land.

VIII

HOSPITAL ECONOMICS COURSE, TEACHERS' COLLEGE.

VIII

HOSPITAL ECONOMICS COURSE, TEACHERS COLLEGE.*

THE Constitution of this Association as originally adopted, recognizes four classes of members, viz: Active, associate, honorary and corresponding members.

In the records of the Annual Meeting of 1896 will be found a report by a special committee on "Eligibility for Membership," the discussion that followed, and the action of the meeting upon that report. Last year another committee was appointed to formulate the necessary changes with a view to a still further amendment. "I think it is in the mind of this Association that we shall have some standard and we are now trying to make a standard. But the question that has lately forced itself upon me is, "Are we working towards the true standard, when we regard as a passport for membership in our Association the position held, rather than the quality of training and education of the woman who holds it. It is true we

* Superintendents' Society, Toronto, 1898.

127

require that "members shall be graduates in good
and regular standing from training schools connected with incorporated general hospitals giving not less
than a two years' course of instruction." So far as
this requirement goes we all meet on common ground,
but we diverge the moment the kind of hospital position held is taken into consideration and on this
basis forthwith are divided into active, associate and
visiting members. It does not seem to me that this
is exactly fair or just to the women who have not
been fortunate enough to secure appointments in
large training schools or who for good reasons may
prefer to do their work in the smaller hospitals,
and hold in them positions that are often just as
responsible, if not more so, than the corresponding
ones in some of the larger institutions. Because a
trained nurse remains in a smaller hospital it does
not signify that she is not just as capable, interested
and progressive in her work as her friend of the larger
school. Besides, on this continent of frequent changes,
it may be the case that we are here to-day and gone
to-morrow, so that the more prominent positions may
at any time be filled by the women from smaller
schools. Would it not seem, therefore, that all other
things being equal, the truer standard must be found
in the qualification of the woman to hold the posi-

tion of a superintendent. This standard once established we could all meet on an equal footing as active members of our Association, equally interested in all that pertains to the best interests of our common work, no matter what position we may hold.

But apart from any question relating to our Association there are other and perhaps stronger reasons why there should be special qualifications required of a woman who would assume so responsible a position as that of a superintendent and teacher in the profession of nursing. Many of us here to-day are the product of the pioneer schools, graduates of years ago when there was more scrubbing required of the pupil-nurse and when less systematic teaching in the theory and practice of nursing was obtainable than is the case to-day. The graduates of these original schools were bound to be the superintendents of all the many other schools that so rapidly sprang into existence, so that we find the pupils of yesterday not infrequently the superintendents of to-day, although, unlike Minerva, they did not spring full grown, armed at every point, ready to do battle in their new work. On the contrary our experience has been won by hard and persistent work—just how hard is only known to each one of us—and the advancements we have made, the improvements we have helped to bring about for the schools of the present day are the result not so much of what we were taught as of what we were *not taught*. Nor need it necessarily reflect upon us to concede that while we were reaching the present measure of our knowledge, our lack of experience was having its daily effect upon those about us, upon the pupils we were instructing, the hospitals we were caring for, and even upon the patients. And this still holds true to a certain extent with every graduate nurse who becomes a superintendent, for as yet there are no special advantages offered to a woman who is desirous of fitting herself to become a superintendent of a training school for nurses. Her principal opportunity is through the experience she gains as a head nurse and in a few instances from such extra training as she has received while acting as an assistant superintendent.

We all recognize that the position of superintendent of nurses requires a woman of executive ability, education, tact, refinement and keen perceptions, and that in addition to these she should have had a thorough all round training in every practical detail of nursing, as well as a thorough course in the theory of her work. But a woman may have all this and still be at a disadvantage when she undertakes her first school for the simple reason that she does not necessarily know the best methods of presenting to others or of teaching her subjects. A sound personal knowledge is a good foundation, but it is quite another matter to be able to impart that knowledge in such a way that it is presented in the best form to the pupil. It is generally conceded by instructors in other kinds of schools that in addition to the diploma secured, it is necessary for those who intend to teach to have a further course in a school of pedagogy or in a normal school, where they may supplement the knowledge they have acquired by learning the principles and the best methods of teaching and how to apply them. Why should not this hold equally well with a woman who elects to become a teacher in a school for nurses? It is one thing to graduate as a trained nurse but quite another thing to enter upon the duties and responsibilities of a training school without a thorough and proper grounding in the management of such work. The woman who lacks this part of her education is placed at a disadvantage from which she cannot recover for some little time.

There are already training schools for teachers established in this country, notably one just recently affiliated with Columbia University, N. Y. Why should not we take advantage of them? For undoubtedly courses could be arranged by which the special requirements of our teachers could be met. The practical requirements we should of course continue to take care of ourselves, but in the theory and didactic part these training schools could supply much which cannot be easily acquired elsewhere.

One of the individual and collective objects of this society is to leave the work of nursing in a better condition than we found it and I think that we may congratulate ourselves upon some of our results. We have thus far worked to some purpose and our time, energy and money have not been expended in vain. Until this year our attention has been chiefly devoted to the interests of the nurses and the work in general, but as at this meeting the subject of ''The Superintendent of the Training School'' is to be under discussion why should we not go a step further and discuss the actual making of the superintendent, *i. e.*, both educational and practical, and her special qualifications? The Society is strong enough and representative enough to initiate the establishment of a Central Board of Examiners whose duty it would be to map out a schedule of requirements for trained nurses who wish to become superintendents of training schools. Besides passing a satisfactory examination in subjects decided upon by this Board, it should be required that a certain length of time should have been spent in some specified training school for teachers, for instruction in the theory of teaching before the successful candidate is entitled to receive a special certificate declaring her fitness to take the position of a superintendent of nurses. It should be the privilege of any graduate nurse whether from a large or small school to come up for these examinations provided she be properly endorsed by her school, and in some instances where a graduate from a smaller school showed general capability and marked ability in her studies, arrangements might be made to afford her additional advantages for work in any branches of practical nursing in which she might still be lacking.

Again, we have discussed the problem of a uniform curriculum. A careful perusal of the able paper presented last year by Miss MeKecknie on ''What has been accomplished in the direction of a uniform curriculum'' will show how far our efforts in this direction still fall short. Would not uniformity in the matter of training teachers make this a natural result in the future work of training schools? It would undoubtedly also be the means of bringing us into closer touch with the smaller hospitals and training schools, and put our work as a society on broader and more uniform lines.

These suggestions have been advanced this year with the hope that the members would give them their careful cansideration and perhaps see their way to appointing a committee to look into the matter more thoroughly and present a plan in detail for the carrying out of some such scheme at not a very distant day.

I am aware that to place our members upon an equal footing would necessitate a complete revision of the Constitution, but this is a mere detail in comparison with the improvements that would result from the establishment of the best tests in deciding upon the suitability of candidates for membership. Can we find any better standard than the educational qualifications?

REPORT ON HOSPITAL ECONOMICS COURSE.

IX

REPORT ON HOSPITAL ECONOMICS COURSE.*

A S chairman of the education committee I regret
to state that we are not as yet prepared to make
a report as a committee, not having been able to hold
one committee meeting, owing to the great distances
that separated us. In September I went to see Miss
Snively, who suggested that I should formulate any
suggestions that I had to offer, and to present them
in writing to the other members of the committee.
This was done and the report I now present was sent
to each member of the committee, but owing to stress
of work the other members did not offer any criticisms. I was able to see Miss Nutting personally three
times and to talk over the proposed plan. It may
be of interest to know what steps led up to the report
about to be presented. In my paper on ''Hospital
Economics Course, Teachers College. I contend that
the qualification for membership in this Society should
be on an educational basis, and in carrying out the
further suggestions in that paper various normal
schools for pedagogy were written to, their methods

---

* Sixth Annual Convention Superintendents' Society, New
York, 1899.

considered. Professors of pedagogy were also interviewed, but nothing was found by any of these means to be practical enough to meet our wants. An appointment was next arranged with the dean of the Teacher's College, which is affiliated with Columbia University, New York City. The visit to the college and the interview were both profitable and encouraging. The college seemed to offer the possibilities of meeting in a practical manner our requirements. At a second interview on the next day Miss Nutting was present. The summer was spent in going over carefully the courses in the college announcement and formulating and adjusting to it our own particular department, and the plan evolved was submitted to Dean Russell at an autumn meeting. After another careful revision the schedule was submitted at a final meeting in December to Miss Kinney, Professor of Domestic Science in the college. Miss Nutting and myself were present at this meeting. The final plan was then drawn up in due form and a copy was sent to each member of the committee. The plan is as follows:

That the Superitnendents' Society appoint a Board of Examiners of experienced superintendents, whose duties are to receive the names of all candidates for the teachers' course, and to endorse them. They decide upon their qualifications as practical trained nurses, examine their certificates, and receive a full statement from the superintendent of the school from which they graduated as to the candidate's qualifications to become a superintendent. In addition to these requirements the Board would require that the candidate enter the Teachers' College for the full term of eight months, and that she will either before or after this term spend from three to four months in doing private duty. Then after this year of extra preparation, having passed the required examination satisfactorily, she should be granted a certificate as a qualified superintendent for a training school for nurses or hospital, such certificate to be signed by the Dean of the Teachers' College and the Board of Examiners. It is desirable that candidates take this course *before* becoming head-nurses. Afterward, and while waiting for appointments, if they can act as head-nurses in the wards of general hospitals from three to six months, so much the better. The average cost for each pupil will be about $400 for the eight months. This includes board, laundry and tuition.

The following table gives in brief the schedule of study suggested, and the following pages contain merely a more detailed description of each course. The course in domestic science would be adapted to the purpose of the work. In general, the course named in the table would be the same as those regularly given in the Teachers' College, except that the course in methods of teaching would be given especially for nurses.

For the course in Hospital Economics it would be necessary to have a trained nurse in charge who has had the necessary experience and qualifications. It is supposed that the three to four months' private duty would enable the candidate to meet nearly all the expense of the college course, in addition to the experience which would be gained at private duty.

The college is splendid. The atmosphere purely educational. I am sure any candidate would find the extra time and money well expended. In regard to Miss Riddle's paper of last year on ''Uniformity in Curriculum,'' her suggestions have been embodied so far as possible in the uniform curriculum as outlined in the course. It is to be hoped by this method that eventually we would attain uniformity in curriculum and training school methods which would make the standing of a trained nurse practically the same from any training school in the country connected with a general hospital. Finally, in the course of time we might be able to supply thoroughly trained superintendents to take charge of the small hospitals and training schools, such superintendents to be entitled to hold active membership in the Superintendents' Society.

X

SOME OF THE LESSONS OF THE LATE WAR AND THEIR BEAR- ING UPON TRAINED NURSING.

X

SOME OF THE LESSONS OF THE LATE WAR AND THEIR BEARING UPON TRAINED NURSING.*

THE pleasure and gratitude with which I accepted, last year, the honor you conferred upon me in again electing me your president, had several sources. Your action testified to your confidence in my efforts in behalf of the Association during the first year of its existence; it showed your willingness to allow the older blood of the pioneers to mingle actively with that of the fresher and later element, and, moreover, emphasized the fact that "once a trained nurse always a trained nurse," and that, though married, a trained nurse need not necessarily be laid on the shelf, but may continue to feel that she still has important duties and obligations toward the profession of which she remains an active life member. Finally, I accept with thankfulness the privilege of assisting in directing a little further the steps at organization which your delegates of last year outlined. The one lion in my path to be dreaded was the obligation laid upon me of making another address; it

---

* Second Annual Convention, Associated Alumnae of Nurses. New York, 1899.

seemed to me all I could possibly have to say had
been said at our first annual meeting. Time, however, has shown me that I need not have faced my
lion so hurriedly, for the year has given me ready to
hand a theme of such deep interest, that in it I shall
hope to find my inspiration to enable me to place it
in some of its bearings clearly before you.

Two events have occurred during the past year,
both of unusual interest to nurses: the first connected
in large part with the past, the other of vital significance for the future of our profession. On March
6th, 1898, a large gathering of trained nurses, physicians and laymen was held in New York, to celebrate
the close of the first quarter of a century of trained
nursing in the United States of America. The year
was also marked by the demand, for the first time,
for the services of trained nurses to meet the emergencies of war. I ask you to allow me, at the risk of
repeating some things which have been said last year,
for a few moments to look back over the past twenty-
five years, because I believe that by so doing I shall
be able to put before you more clearly certain phases
of the second and more important subject of my address, namely, What lessons has the late war taught
us, and what bearing or influence may it have upon
trained nursing in the future?

It is usually the custom with all well-regulated
business concerns to take account, at stated times, of

their affairs; to go over their past records, and find
out just how much has been accomplished, and how
much, if anything, stands to their credit for the future. As we have just rounded off our first quarter
of a century, it is then in order for us to re-read our
records, and see how we have fared during that time,
and in how far the outlook for the future is hopeful.
The trained nurse is a distinctly modern product.
Twenty-five years ago we find her just starting out
on her career, without antecedents, without experience, with all before her, and all to learn. Her cre-
dentials had to be of her own making, her professional standing had to be evolved; she had to establish her own traditions, and in all these undertakings
she had to maintain her own personal and professional dignity. She has, however, never lacked for
friends, for here in New York the seed was sown by
women for women and for the good of suffering humanity. And these founders of a new guild for women have stood through these first years ever loyal
and true to watch over the best interests of the young
plant, proping where necessary, pruning judiciously,
and ever giving wise and friendly counsel. So long
as the success or failure of the trained nurse was an
open question, her development was naturally slow,
but after the first few years, when graduates began
to increase in numbers and the value of their work
had been manifest in the hospital and home, we find

more branches beginning to shoot out, and more training schools springing into existence. In the past ten years more especially, there has been a not altogether healthy overgrowth; the increase has been almost alarming, and there are now to be found all sorts and conditions of hospitals and training schools, with the result that the country has been flooded with a very nondescript class of women, all bearing the title of trained nurse, the term standing for all grades of training and all grades of women. As a natural consequence, the public has freely offered its criticisms, various and varied in character, upon the trained nurse, the good and bad having to bear their share equally of praise or blame. Here, then, was the first problem to confront us—the rapid increase in quantity without a corresponding improvement in quality—and as this discrepancy became more and more apparent, the older and better known schools, with the instinct of self-preservation, began to draw more closely within themselves, trusting in their own irreproachable names to protect their graduates, with the result that the members of one school were led to hold themselves severely aloof from those of another. Fortunately, this narrow and selfish policy could not last long. Gradually but forcibly it was borne in upon the minds of the older and more experienced that in this way did not lie success and advancement; that nurses could not afford to be narrow and self-seeking, and that to attain to a fixed high standard in our work, to overcome the evils that were increasing, and to collect our scattered forces, we must have unity of purpose and centralization of means. As an expression of this growing conviction, a Congress of Nurses was held in Chicago, in 1893. During this meeting, a number of superintendents, feeling the obligations resting upon them, either as a reward or penance for being many of them pioneers among nurses, and all of them representing most of the large schools in the country, met together to discuss ways and means by which some of these problems would be met, and some of the evils overcome. This conference resulted in the formation of the American Society of Superintendents of Training Schools for Nurses. Beginning with a membership of 18, the roll gradually increased, until it now includes over 100 members, or practically the heads of all the best training schools in the country. During its five years of work it has labored faithfully to lay a solid foundation upon which a standard for nurses might be built—a standard that all high-minded, earnest nurses would be proud to help to maintain, and that would attract to the work desirable women. From the first the society was impressed with the fact that only by the nurses themselves could such a standard be created and sustained, and, before anything like a professional status could be hoped for, an *esprit de corps* must be established among graduates of the same school, with a drawing together in their own work and home interests. It was felt that this sentiment, once actively aroused, an interest in the larger affairs and problems of nurses as a class would naturally follow. The fact that in this short time alumnæs have been organized in almost every training school, both large and small, that the Associated Alumnæ is just completing its second year with a membership of 26 alumnæs, representing about 2,500 nurses, and that this year many small general schools will be admitted into associated membership, is a convincing proof that trained nurses require a fixed standard, that they are alive to their responsibilities as professional women, and realize that they have a definite position to maintain. And so we close this brief *resume* of the first quarter of a century of our history, with a knowledge that our chief weakness during these years has come from the rapid increase in numbers, from the want of a professional and educational standard, and from the scattering of our forces from lack of organization and of working together in our common interests. But there is nothing to be despondent over, and much ground for encouragement. We are fortunate in having discovered our weakest points at so early a period in our career. Our strength in all that tends toward bettering the work of the trained nurse is in a fair way to increase.

If our efforts toward organization are still incomplete, a fair beginning has been made, and, at least, we are free from many factions, with their working at cross-purposes, for which we may be deeply thankful. Steps have been taken to decrease the quantity of graduates, as well as to improve the standard, by increasing the term of instruction from two to three years. There is also more uniformity in candidates, requirements, and more system in our methods of instruction. "Well begun is half done," and, at least, we may congratulate ourselves that we have made a good beginning.

And now, let us turn and look a little way into the future, and mark what it may hold for us in the way of new work, responsibilities and obligations. Nor have we far to look, for right on the threshold we are confronted by a problem that holds grave results and responsibilities for trained nurses. In my last year's address, I mentioned some of the branches of work, in addition to hospital and private nursing, that have been opened up to the trained nurse, all evidences of the growing place which the world is ready to give her as she shows her fitness for it. To these was unexpectedly added another in the demand and need for her services during the late war.

Last spring, when the possibilities of war menaced the nation, individual nurses expressed their willingness to give their services, if needed, in the military hospitals, and when war was actually declared, the number of volunteers was greatly increased. But, unfortunately, trained nurses were not the only women thus impelled, for applications and offers to do army nursing began to pour into the Surgeon-General's office from all manner of women, from the well-meaning "born nurse," the enthusiastic patriot, from sisterhoods and from adventuresses, as well as from the cream and slum of trained nurses. Just about this time the Associated Alumnæ was holding its first annual meeting in New York, and one of the first acts its delegates had the privilege of performing was to offer the services of representative trained nurses, as a body, to the government, to do its army nursing. This step was taken because the delegates were fully impressed with the fact that nursing in the army is of the greatest importance to the country, and that here, if anywhere, incompetence and want of system would be productive of the greatest harm, not only in the immediate present, but for the future of many valuable lives. You all know how nobly our volunteer forces behaved, but the backbone of our military and naval resources lay in the trained men —the trained members of our army and navy. In the same way it was only logical to assume that the backbone of nursing should be found in trained women, who for years had made this their profession. These, it was thought, should form a nucleus around which could be built up a proper system and efficiency in the nursing. I would particularly insist that the Associated Alumnæ of trained nurses did not desire that all the nurses for the army should be selected from their ranks; what they did ask, was that the service should be organized from a strictly business standpoint, and that, for nursing, trained women should be selected, and that each individual nurse should be chosen only after affording some guarantee that she had been fitted by a proper training for the work in hand. The following telegram was therefore dispatched to the Surgeon-General:

"April 28, 1898.

"To the Hon. Secretary of War, Washington, D. C.:

"The Associated Alumnæ of Trained Nurses of the United States and Canada, including 2,000 graduates of twenty-four training schools, offer their services for any work which the Medical Department of the army may demand of them, in connection with the war with Spain.

"By direction of the delegates now in session in New York City."

But not receiving any reply, and believing that a personal interview, explaining the number and standing of these nurses, would result in the acceptance of their services, the president and vice-president of the Association went down to Washington and had a personal interview with the Surgeon-General. But their mission was a failure, as they were told that the nursing department had been given into the charge of the Daughters of the American Revolution, with a woman doctor as director. Visions of what splendid systematic work might be done if the nursing might only be in the hands of the nurses themselves, supplemented by the extra supplies so generously provided by the D. A. R., the Red Cross and other societies, floated before us, but it was not to be. The story of the summer's campaign is familiar to many of us. The chaos and confusion that reigned supreme at first, owing to the suddenness and greatness of the emergency, was intensified and prolonged by the lack of experience on the part of those into whose hands the work was entrusted. This and the appointments made from all the varieties of women mentioned above resulted in much bad nursing, a worse morale, and in a total lack of standard or system. How long such a condition would have continued to exist, it is hard to say, had not the situation been saved by the assistance and admirable work rendered by the Red Cross Auxiliary, No. 3.

A brief word in explanation of these Red Cross Auxiliaries. They did not form a permanent part of the American National Red Cross Society, but were made up of a number of patriotic men and women, who organized for the purpose of raising funds to assist the government in any way they might, in relieving the needs and suffering of the sick soldiers. That they might do this the more effectually, they offered themselves as auxiliaries to the Red Cross Society already in the field. After the emergency of the war was over, they disbanded. Auxiliary No. 3 was organized for the express purpose of ''supplying and maintaining trained nurses in army hospitals.'' Too much cannot be said in praise of the work they accomplished, hampered as they were by being only auxiliaries and not the controlling head. It was through this Auxiliary that the best nursing was done; they put themselves at once in touch with trained nurses of experience and ability, and continued to co-operate with them to the end. But with lack of experience at the head, and with nurses recruited from a variety of sources, there was necessarily much chaff among the wheat. A certain amount of good nursing was done, but not half of what could have been accomplished with proper management. Protest upon protest has come to my ears from the nurses and others competent to judge of these matters, and I have received numerous letters, asking if some better condition of army nursing could not be established, and insisting upon the absolute necessity of inaugurating a better system, with more order, discipline, and, consequently, better work. Many good nurses who went into military hospitals during the summer returned home again, not because they were not willing to put up with physical discomforts, but because they could not tolerate the lack of discipline and the looseness of work and conduct, and because they could not conscientiously serve under the young, inexperienced and indiscreet women often placed over them.

Do not understand me as saying that all the hospitals and nurses were unsatisfactory, for just when the stress of work was greatest, the superintendents of experience and ability, with their nurses, chosen by the Red Cross Auxiliary No. 3, did much to minimize the lamentable state of affairs which had existed up to that time. Certainly, then, one of the important lessons to be learned from the war is that the nursing system in the army, as it existed during the war and as it exists at the present day, leaves much to be desired. Sad experience has shown us that those who do the country's fighting and suffer for their flag, do not, in the hour of need, receive such good care as many a worthless tramp is thought to be entitled to in a civil hospital. At least, let the mothers, wives and sisters of the soldiers have the satisfaction of feeling that their loved ones, when wounded or sick, shall have the best nursing procurable. And if women are acknowledged to be the best nurses of the sick in times of peace, why not also in war? Our army surgeons are taken from among the graduates of our best medical schools; our army nurses should be taken from our best training schools for nurses.

But in order to have such a service ready to be utilized in time of war or emergency, the work of organization must be intelligently done in the time of peace. No one will dispute the fact that the country must have always at its command a regular army of trained soldiers. Why is it not, then, just as logical to keep ever ready a standing army of trained nurses, who come up to a fixed standard, and that the highest in every way? The day for the volunteer nurse, the born nurse, and the enthusiastic, patriotic women to do army nursing has gone by, just as the old and often haphazard methods in hygiene and surgery have given place to modern scientific surgery and medicine, the result of investigation and training. Nor can the nurses who intelligently put into execution the methods and orders of the scientific physician be made in a day. As a member of the House of Representatives very aptly said: ''The work is a work of their own; it cannot be done by others.'' There is plenty of work for the energy and generosity of such fine organizations as the D. A. R. and the National Red Cross Society, and our impulse has been and always will be to lend a helping hand to them when opportunity affords. But this one particular branch must be left to trained nurses, and if we are to be held responsible for the results of the nursing, the power of making a proper selection of women for the work should rest in our own hands. Only then can our failures be justly cast in our teeth.

But as representatives of the trained nurses of this country, we have felt that before submitting our views to the consideration of the government, it was necessary to make sure that they had the endorsement of the people at large, and especially those who had studied the question of nursing in the army. While considering how to reach this opinion, which, judging from numerous articles in the daily papers and in the magazines, was certainly widespread, and while debating how we might get in touch with this friendly aid, we learned to our joy that among the men and women who had so generously given of their time, strength and money to aid in providing skilled nursing during all the long summer, there were not a few who held the same conviction as the nurses themselves, and who, anxious that some permanent good should result from the summer's work and experience, were willing to continue their aid and work for this end when once they were assured that the nurses were willing to undertake permanently this new field of nursing. No time was lost in assuring them of our readiness, and the result was that a meeting was called in New York, in December, 1898, under the auspices of the Associated Alumnæ of

Trained Nurses, to confer with those interested as to the proper steps to be taken. It was unanimously decided that a bill should be prepared and presented to Congress to provide for the establishment of women nurses in military hospitals. To formulate this bill and to secure its success, a joint committee was formed, composed of women prominent among those who have deserved well of their country, a certain number of trained nurses from among those who had been in active service during the war, or of experience as superintendents of nurses, whose time and services were available for bringing the matter to the notice of the authorities at Washington. After the formation of this committee, any active part the Associated Alumnæ took as a body, was at an end, since the committee felt that in any bill on army nursing trained nurses should be considered as a professional body, and that in its enactments, no exclusive society should be recognized. In drawing up the bill, the endeavor was made to embody all the essentials that world assure a high order of nursing. It is, indeed, most important that the first step should be carefully taken, in order not to bring the whole subject of women nurses in the army into unmerited disrepute. The following statement, read in Washington at one of the meetings held in favor of the bill, admirably expresses what the committee had in mind, and will convey to your minds their views far better than could any words of mine:

February 2nd, 1899.

The views of the chiefs of the large training schools for women nurses, and of the ladies who are especially interested in this movement, is that it is a matter of very great importance to select proper women for the first appointments as nurses in the army service, under this or any other bill.

It is not merely that the persons so selected should be able to pass an ordinary examination to determine the capacity of the trained nurse, such as might possibly be provided by the Civil Service Commission, but they should be persons who are selected for their tact and discretion, and, to a considerable extent, for business capacity, and that the only persons who can obtain perfectly reliable information upon these points are the heads of some of the more important training schools, or persons who have been connected with them.

The feeling of those who are urging this bill is that it is a reasonably certain way to secure for the army the kind of women nurses whom it is so desirable to obtain, and while the method proposed may not be precisely in accordance with military precedents, they feel bound to urge it, in view of the great importance of the matter.

The ordinary method would be, of course, to provide that these nurses should be selected by the Surgeon-General of the Army, which would mean by a board to be organized by him. But no board which he could organize, composed of members of the medical staff, could by any possibility obtain the information as to qualifications, outside of the purely technical qualifications, above referred to, and it would find itself unable to judge of the relative merits of the various testimonials and certificates with which it is quite certain that every candidate who came before such a board, would be amply provided. Unless we can make sure that the right kind of women are selected in the beginning to take charge of the introduction of women nurses into the army, we think it doubtful whether it would be worth while to attempt to introduce women nurses at all at the present time, for a very few women, having more zeal than discretion, and not able to cope with the various petty difficulties which are sure to occur at first, will be likely to bring the whole subject of women nurses in the army into unmerited disrepute.

It follows, therefore, that the standard for these first nurses to be appointed must necessarily be high. Our object should be to secure women who can manage, or, if necessary, instruct, less qualified nurses, whom it may be necessary to employ hereafter. It would be the greatest possible mistake to employ any but the very best nurses to begin this work.

The fate of the bill still lies in the future, as there was not time for it to come before the Senate at the last session. The work done for it so far goes to show how warmly the public, as well as the government, approve of it, for it has already received a majority vote in Congress, which undoubtedly would have been larger had there been a clear understanding in the minds of all the representatives as to some of its details. There was unexpected opposition on the part of the National Red Cross Society, whose privileges and work we had not any thought of interfering with; on the contrary, we had hoped, by our own organization, to render their work in the future much more efficient, for the reason that they would no longer have to depend upon auxiliaries to supply them with nurses in times of emergency. Again, it would be a mistake to assume that the bill would debar any Red Cross nurse from serving, for its measures allow for the acceptance of any or all trained nurses, provided they enter the army nursing corps in the prescribed way, and can meet the requirements necessary for a fixed standard of ability, health, education, and morals.

And now, what is the duty of each individual, right-minded, trained nurse in regard to this bill? It is that she shall give it her loyal support in all legitimate ways known to her until it becomes law. It will be presented to Congress at its next session, and between now and then she should work for it untiringly, for, if successful, it means that the professional standing and standard for the trained nurse will have been won, for we shall have the seal and the recognition of the nation stamped upon us, which should incite us to greater efforts, to prove ourselves worthy of so great an honor and trust. At the present time there is no modern system of army nursing in any country, and it should be our pride and pleasure to make that of the United States one that would be an object-lesson for all countries to follow.

If the bill, however, should fail, then we shall, as a body and as individuals, have a still graver question to face. Shall we be loyal and strong enough to stand by the standard we are striving to make for ourselves, or shall we dissipate our forces and enlist as, in the old way, under any society, under any leadership, and with any kind of nurses? The past twenty-five years has shown a curious apathy on the part of the trained nurses to take care of their own affairs, and, had we time, I could cite several instances in which outsiders are taking the lead and making a profit, and sometimes their living, out of trained nurses, while the nurses themselves seem content, and forget the best interests of the profession to follow these self-seeking leaders, like sheep. For many the temptation to choose the easier path will be hard to resist, for present remuneration is much more tangible and attractive than a possible future standard. During the war the trained nurse has suffered. She has been called to account, not only for her own faults, but the shortcomings of incompetent amateurs have also been reckoned against her. Can any graduate think it right to help to perpetuate such a reproach by enlisting into any body that lacks a proper organization and a proper standard? Is the mess of pottage worth sacrificing our birthright for? Can we dare to run the risk of making the name of trained nurse more of a reproach than it has been? Remember, ''A motive that gives a sublime rhythm to a woman's life and exalts habit into partnership with the world's highest needs, is not to be had how and where she wills; to know that high initiation she must often tread where it is hard to tread, and feel the chill air, and watch through darkness.'' We need never be afraid that our standard will ever become too exalted, for even with our best efforts there will always be those among us who wear the cap and gown who will bring dishonor upon it sufficient to strike a balance and keep us lowly-minded enough. But how great the dishonor for all of us if we do not try to maintain a good, practical average, at least!

During the past quarter of a century we have unconsciously and independently helped to do much; let us now, realizing our strength, resolve to do more; let us, by being more closely united as a body, become a more powerful factor for good. While working as individuals in other organizations, for their many and varied objects, let us be bound by one common tie to this, our profession; and no matter how great may be the temptations to divert our strength from its legitimate field, let us hold steadfast and thus win confidence and respect which must be jealously guarded and steadily increased by the faithful loyalty and personal interest of every woman within the ranks, each and all content to put into our work only the highest and best we have to give. Remember, we are the history-makers of trained nurses. Let us see to it that we work so as to leave a fair record as the inheritance of those who come after us, one which may be to them an inspiration to even better efforts, instead of a regret or a reproach. It rests with ourselves entirely just how honored, how useful, and what place this nursing work shall hold in the world. Certain it is, that if we do not get credit for our successful efforts, we shall inevitably incur reproach for whatever may sully the work of our profession. Whatever be the result of our efforts, whatever the verdict of the present generation, or of posterity, let each of us see to it that we make ourselves safe from the pangs of self-reproach. Then, and only then, if the consciousness of duty done be our only reward, it will suffice.

XI

STATE REGISTRATION.

STATE REGISTRATION.*

O NLY once during the twelve months is it our privilege to meet together as a corporate body to deal with the common affairs of our common work, to take counsel, as wisely as we may, how we may improve and further that work by mutual and organized efforts, and at the same time strengthen those ties which bind us together as individual workers and as members of a profession, which in a little over twenty-five years has grown, as it were, from a small seed to a mighty tree whose branches spread widely and in many direction. To this yearly gathering also are brought the suggestions of individual members and of individual alumnæ associations to receive the consideration and attention of the representatives of the whole body, who deliberate upon them and take such action as seems best. The result of these deliberations, together with the substance of the papers read and of the ensuing discussions, are reported to the several alumnæ by their delegates, and moreover are printed in detail in the annual report, which is circulated through the proper channels, so that it comes within the reach of even the most remote mem-

---

* Associated Alumnae of Nurses, New York, 1900.

ber, supplying her, we trust, with fresh food for thought and a new stimulus for the work of the next year.

It would seem, therefore, advisable that we should make use of this annual opportunity to hold a general review of our forces, so that utilizing what we can learn from the retrospect we may be the better able to deal with the present and receive a clearer understanding as regards the future. Our looking backward does not as yet give us much ground to cover, since this is only the third time we have met together, and our combined deliberations cover only two years of work. But even in this short time we have been brought face to face with circumstances which are of deep import to all nurses, and which have caused the need for concentrated interest and work to be keenly felt. To those of our members to whom the benefits to be derived from organization were perhaps not yet clear, I feel sure that certain events of the past two years have shown the imperative need for organization, so that I trust that this question may be regarded as permanently settled. Indeed to our cost we now know that the concentration of our forces came too late by at least a year, for one can hardly doubt that the nursing of our soldiers during the Spanish-American war would naturally have fallen into our hands, had our professional organization been completed earlier. If this had been done, our capacity

to meet properly so important a crisis would have
been better understood and appreciated, with the result that not only would our soldiers have received
better nursing, but we ourselves might have been
spared the extra exertion that has been demanded of
us during the past two years in our continued efforts
in supporting the Army Nursing Bill, and at the same
time upholding the honor of our professional status.
It may be, however, as well that we were not successful to begin with, for had honors come to us too
easily, they might possibly have rendered us careless
of our best interests in the future, and the necessity
for absolute loyalty and continued personal effort
might not have been so early impressed upon our
minds with sufficient emphasis. Be that as it may,
the events of the past year have made even the doubt-
ers among us realize that, in a certain sense, the
trained nurse as a unit is nobody; and although at
this writing the success or failure of the Army Nursing Bill is still undecided we may still feel that,
whether we win or lose the cause for this year, we
should be deeply grateful that we were a sufficiently
organized and representative body to be able to unite
in working to uphold and guard our professional hon-
or and its welfare.

In other ways also, there has been a closer drawing together and a broader outlook developed, chiefly
through the efforts of our Educational Committee.

For the purpose of education in various cities, alumnæ members of different schools have met together, and, in accordance with the programme submitted by the Educational Committee, courses of lectures and talks on various topics have been arranged and well attended meetings have been held at the various alumnæ club rooms. Incidentally this exchange of alumnæ courtesies has been the means of stirring up a considerable pride and ambition in individual school alumnæs, and as a result new club houses have been established. These meetings may also be regarded as the forerunners of the local clubs which we shall hope to see begun in the near future.

But no doubt the chief subject that has largely held our interest during the two years past has been army nursing, and the various phases of the problem have been studied by many of us with keen interest. To-day the need for a better organization of the nursing forces on a modern basis in every country is being as plainly demonstrated in South Africa as it was in the late Spanish-American war, although, happily for the sufferers, not to the same painful extent as happened in the case of our own soldiers. But as was only natural, efforts to bring about a better state of affairs at once developed the opposition which is always encountered by work which is healthy and progressive. Fortunately the opposition comes from the outside and is purely commercial; it does not represent any high aims or definite principles; its leaders are not trained nurses, and the success of their projects would mean the complete subjection of trained nurses. We have, therefore, no common ground upon which any compromise can be effected. When trained nurses have demonstrated their inability to look after their own affairs, then and not till then can they permit themselves to be guided and governed by women, whose ruling motive must be a commercial one, as such women cannot appreciate the work to be done or the proper methods for performing it, as can trained nurses themselves.

The growth of our association is steady and encouraging. This year we add five more large schools to our membership and six small general schools will be admitted into associate membership as soon as certain changes in the constitution, which will be made at this meeting, have rendered the step legal. At this meeting also we shall be called upon to consider the question of enlarging our borders in order to admit, on the same footing as alumnæ associations, local associations, some of whose members have not had the opportunity of being connected with alumnæ (in case such associations do not exist in their schools), but who would bring into a local association the same standard as that required by our alumnæs. Each alumnæ has received due notice of the amendment to come up at this meeting, so no doubt you are all conversant with the pros and cons of the question. It is desired that this point shall be settled before we proceed to the formation of state associations, which the various alumnæs of New York purpose to take steps to do very shortly in their state. This will not be the first time the question of local and state associations has come before us for discussion. A large portion of our First Annual Report is made up of papers and discussions upon the subjects of state and local associations. I would strongly recommend each member of this association to provide herself with a copy of the First Annual Report and read and consider carefully the points brought out at our first meeting; if this is done, I am sure the need for such associations will be better understood. At that same meeting a committee was appointed to report upon the formation of local associations. Last year no written report was submitted by that committee, but I should like to quote from the verbal report made by its chairman:

"Not much has been accomplished this year, but there has been a good deal of thinking done. It seems that the time is coming for the forming of local associations, thus uniting those alumnæ associations which are eligible for representation in the national association, and which should include stray graduates of other schools who are in good standing in their own alumnæ associations. It would mean that all the associations and the graduates must be eligible to membership in the national association. I cannot see how local associations could be formed on other lines. But it is evident that that would bar out a great many women who graduated years ago from schools that are not eligible to membership in this association, and yet there is no doubt of the great benefit it would be to these women to work with such local associations. Probably it is those nurses who would be most anxious to attend such meetings and who would derive most benefit from them. I am aware from things that have come to my notice that these should be much more comprehensive than the original idea of the local association. The whole subject is something that has to be considered. No actual work has been done as yet. The question is, how inclusive shall they be?'' This is just the question which we trust our delegates have come prepared to answer and settle at this meeting. It is not one of my duties to instruct you, but I may at least ask you to remember that our object in associating is to advance the interests of the whole *nursing profession* and not merely those of any one association. After deciding upon the formation of local associations we trust steps may very soon be taken to formulate state associations, beginning in all probability with the state of New York.

As many of us know, the question of registration

for trained nurses has been long in our minds, but we were also aware that to advocate legislation for nurses eight or ten years ago would have been to "put the cart before the horse." At that time, no *esprit de corps* existed among the leaders in our schools. Nothing much in the way of systematic teaching was recognized; certainly there was no uniformity in curriculum and not even an attempt at a general education and ethical standard. Among the nurses there was no professional feeling, not even among the graduates of the same school; there was simply nothing organized or professional about us. Collectively we could neither qualify as a profession, a calling, or a trade. For to be a member of a profession implies more responsibility, more serious duties, a higher skill and work demanding a more thorough education than is required in many other vocations in life. But two things more are needful—organization and legislation. A calling, in its accepted sense, implies more exclusively a consecrated religious life, such as that of sisterhoods with their religious restrictions, which are more numerous and exacting than those demanded of the trained nurse; while, on the other hand, a trade is more largely concerned with manual labor. We were, therefore, a most indefinite quantity. How then, could we ask for legislation as a profession, when we did not exist as such? We had, therefore, to know and understand ourselves, in some measure, before we could possibly determine our rightful status. Modern medicine, in requiring of us the professional attributes, has taken the decision out of our hands, and has made trained nursing a profession; but how soon we shall attain to the full profession level depends upon ourselves entirely. Before all, then, it was necessary to organize, and the rapidity and thoroughness with which you went at and accomplished the first steps were truly amazing, and not the least delightful part to witness has been the splendid, broad-minded, liberal spirit with which you have met each other, This passing tribute of pride and pleasure in your achievements may be permitted to one who has watched unceasingly every step in your growth and who knows whereof she speaks. These important phases in development, though comparatively rapid, have followed each other in their natural sequence; as a result there has been no time lost in retracing steps, but a gradual broadening out has been going on as need arose. Thus organization has developed through the Society of Superintendents standing for educational advancement, to the school alumnæs, representing home as well as professional interests, to the national association representing the profession, with its larger life and affairs, and where each alumnæ has equal representation. Furthermore, after this meeting we may hope for the rapid development of local associations, where each nurse, in one state and town to-day and in another far away to-morrow, may still have her recognized place and voice in the affairs of her profession; and finally, before we meet again, we look for the formation of at least one state association, the last link in the chain of organization.

But with the completion of the chain the fulness of time brings us face to face with the vital question of registration for nurses, the foundation for which was laid just seven years ago. State registration is certainly the next and most important step towards achieving a fixed professional standard. According to the Constitution of the United States, an act authorizing registration for the whole profession and country cannot be passed by Congress at Washington, but each state must make its own laws for its own nurses. New York with its local and state associations will become sufficiently representative to ask for legal recognition for trained nurses within its domains. It is only fitting that this state should take the initiative. Its educational institutions are controlled by the University of the State of New York, which does not allow members of any profession to practice in the state until they show proper proofs that they have graduated from some recognized qualified school, and have also passed certain prescribed examinations in the studies taught in these schools. Only to those who satisfy these requirements is a license granted by the regents of the university. If then, similar requirements had to be met by trained nurses, nursing would at once be established on a distinct educational plane. Again, as New York is the home of the mother of training schools in this country, it is but fitting that this state should first receive the crowning glory of the work she so bravely undertook. Nor will the other states lag far behind her in this respect if we may judge by the alacrity with which they followed her lead in establishing schools for nurses. Only by a complete system of registration will it be possible for trained nursing to attain to its full dignity as a recognized profession and obtain permanent reforms. As the matter stands at present, the woman who has spent years of hard work and study in acquiring skill and knowledge as a nurse, on undertaking private nursing, finds at once that she is classed on a level with all sorts and grades of so-called trained nurses; nor has she any redress. She is expected to work side by side with the uncertified hospital nurse, who has been dismissed for cause before the expiration of her term as a student, with the half trained nurse from the specialty hospitals, with the nurse who has received the kind of instruction that makes her dangerous, with the adventuress, and the amateur—women masquerading as nurses, a matter of uniforms with no knowledge behind them —with the second-year hospital pupil sent out during the time that should have been devoted to her education, to earn money for the institution. Is it to be wondered at that with such a levelling, with the competent confused with the incompetent in the eyes of the public, that the severe and continual criticism should fall upon the just as well as upon the unjust and that the nursing profession should suffer for the sins and shortcomings of those who should not be ranked as belonging to it. Our sympathies are divided between a long-suffering and much sinned against public and the genuine trained nurse. Such anomalous conditions have gone far towards bringing private duty into bad odor and as a result many of our best graduates prefer to remain in hospitals, at a much less income, because there they hold a definite recognized professional status, since in all hospitals worthy of the name the authorities recognize the necessity and importance of having trained nurses in charge of the nursing department, and the staff is made up either of graduates or pupils, no room or place remaining for nondescripts.

But with registration this unfortunate condition of things will be changed; the professional status of the trained nurse will be defined no less sharply than that of the physician or of the lawyer. By these means also the public would be provided with a distinguishing mark whereby they could know whether any given nurse has been properly trained, and is a suitable person to take charge of the sick; whereas in the absence of a public registry or of a physician to make the selection they are left without any guarantee of the efficiency of the various candidates. Again, since the medical profession must always wish to secure for their patients the best care, it will undoubtedly heartily endorse this further effort to increase and improve the efficiency of the nursing service. Lastly, as regards training schools themselves, the introduction of a legalized registration would naturally stimulate both schools and graduates to reach the required educational standard. Each school would be obliged to give the pupils a sufficiently thorough instruction in the theory and practice of nursing as would enable them to pass the examination prescribed by law, and obtain the certificate, which would authorize them to practice as trained nurses. These examinations could be conducted by properly qualified boards, the members of which would be largely drawn from those among the ranks of the trained nurses who have had special experience in such matters; who know what good nursing is, how it should be taught, and what standard is desirable and at the same time attainable.

Of course such a law would not be retroactive and would not affect graduate nurses, who were already in the field, beyond requiring them to present their diplomas and applying for registration.

With this final step in our professional organization accomplished, we are then ready to set to work to some purpose to define our ethical code which belongs to the other side of nursing—the corrective of a too pronounced professional attitude, and which in its fulfilment rounds off our work.

Although we are nearing the completion of the last links of our national organization there are still others to be forged, by which we hope to unite ourselves in professional bonds with those of our own guild in other countries and become identified with woman's work at large all over the world, thus gaining additional breadth and strength for our own more specialized efforts. Last year you may remember, we were proffered the privilege of membership in the International Council of Women; this year we have a similar invitation from the International Council of Nurses, which is one of the outcomes of last year's meeting, and which in itself goes to show that American nurses are by no means alone in feeling the need for organization. Indeed the work that nurses are achieving along these lines in other countries makes interesting and inspiring reading and brings home to each one of us convincingly the importance of personal loyalty, personal interest and personal work, without which we can never hope to attain the full measure of success. At our first annual meeting Miss Dolliver put the case exactly when she said, "So long as there is one graduate who is not with us, we are weak by so much as her mind, character and influence are valued at.'' If we do not take care of our own affairs, rest assured that outsiders will undertake the task for us to our everlasting undoing and to the detriment of the public, whose sick we have the privilege of ministering to.

Whether we shall take up or lay aside our professional responsibilities is not a matter of choice, but a question of duty and conscience. Do you think it right that any one of us, who has come to a clear understanding of the seriousness and importance of nursing work should go her separate way and take her own ease and pleasure while there is even one human life imperiled for the want of good nursing? Can we be still and let things just take their own way, so long as the stamp of mediocrity marks a work to which should be given the best and highest that the hands, hearts and minds of women can bring to it? This is no work that can be taken up lightly or laid aside carelessly by the first-comer, but one that should be entrusted only to women, each one of whom should be ordained a priestess, as it were, before she presumes to enter into the temple to perform her ministries unto sick and suffering humanity.

XII

WOMEN ON HOSPITAL BOARDS.

WOMEN ON HOSPITAL BOARDS.*

S O much has already been said about the advantages and disadvantages of putting the administration of hospitals in the hands of boards composed
of women as well as men, that at first sight any additional remarks would hardly seem to be required.
Nevertheless, the whole subject is one about which
nurses, whether they be superintendents or others
occupied inside or outside of hospitals, should take
pains carefully to inform themselves, for opportunities come to many of us when the right kind of knowledge would be of much value in helping either the individual or the public to reach correct conclusions
concerning this and other questions in which similar
principles are involved. For these reasons, this brief
paper that I have had the honor to prepare for the
Congress, is devoted to the consideration of our attitude of mind as a profession towards the appointment
of women on hospital boards, and an endeavor has
been made to place a true value upon woman's services in such work, to consider some of the ways in
which a proper selection may be made, and some of
the methods of organizing her work by which the most

---

* International Convention of Nurses, Buffalo, 1901.

effective service may be rendered while harmony is preserved. In taking an honest vote of our position towards the subject, judging from opinions freely expressed in private and from our negative attitude in reference to it in public, it is safe to say that in all probability, superintendents would be almost unanimously in favor of working in hospitals where women are not represented on the managing boards. This feeling is partly due simply to the traditional belief in woman's incompatibility to work with women—and we know how slowly all fixed traditions die—and partly to the fact that in some instances this incompatibility has been a matter of personal experience, which has been swiftly carried from one to another, and has not failed to leave a prejudice in the minds of every hearer. For less reason the feeling is usually shared in by the staff of hospital nurses, being founded not so much upon any special comments they may have heard passed upon lady managers, or upon any particular reasoning on their own part, but being the natural outcome of a certain unsympathetic tone respecting the matter that pervades the hospital, fostered, it may be, by the unspoken but negative attitude on the part of the superintendent, and occasionally by the thoughtless remarks of inexperienced, unthinking members of the hospital staff, who regard with suspicion the possibility of outside interference in their own particular province. This conception might be expressed in words somewhat as follows: ''Visiting ladies are apt to be interfering, opinionated in affairs they cannot know very much about, busy-bodies and stirrers up of trouble. They are therefore to be regarded with suspicion and treated with scant or only forced courtesy.'' That some such feeling pervaded hospitals twenty years ago I can testify, and it seems but yesterday that I recall with what transparent toleration the ladies' visits were received in the wards by the nurses. In my own particular case nothing but good to myself came from the only occasion on which, as a pupil, I encountered one of the lady members of the board. She came behind the screen where I was busy in caring for a patient, and after taking in some of the details, abruptly put the question, ''Can you comb a patient's hair so that it doesn't pull and hurt the patient all the time? There is not one nurse in a hundred who knows how to comb a patient's hair properly.'' She passed on, leaving with me the determination to excel in at least that one point in nursing so that after that time I never arranged a patient's hair without giving special thought to her comfort. As regards superintendents, the true source of their objection lies in the dread that their own ideas and ways may be interfered with or hampered, or that they may be disturbed by constant and untimely visits and by unnecessary solicitations for patients from individual members, or by the board as a whole. To always do our work in our own way may be very pleasant, but where this work has to do so vitally with so many people, both well and ill, and where it is a public trust, the surest sign that we are broadening out with growth in years and experience is evidenced by an ever increasing readiness to give up prejudices and to welcome any arrangement that will help the work on. To do the subject justice, we must in the first place take an absolutely impartial and impersonal view of it. To eliminate the personal equation is very difficult, but this must be done, and only the thought of the benefit that such boards are likely to be to the hospital should be allowed to influence us. In nursing as in any other work the more self is kept in the background, and the more the work and its best interests are made the first thought and consideration, the happier the worker, and the greater the success obtained, for the reason that over-sensitiveness and friction will seldom interfere. Were I to allow the personal sentiment to predominate I should take the side against the election of women to serve on hospital boards, as I did at a time in my hospital career when I certainly was not a fit judge on so important a matter, since I had not yet made a trial of both ways of working. Increasing experience, however, coupled with an unswerving determination to make the best interests of the hospital my first consideration, have led me to alter my former opinion, and I can hardly express myself too strongly in favor of their appointment. This decision is the result of personal experience obtained from various sources. For some years I worked in two of the largest hospitals in the country, where the administration of the hospital and training school in each case was quite distinct, the former being entirely in the hands of men, and the latter in those of women. In a third hospital, the trustees of which are all men, the women formed an auxiliary board, and although giving lavishly of their time and means to procure materials and necessaries generally for the hospital, were not accorded even the right to demand an account of the disposition of the abundant supplies provided by them. In another large hospital, in which I was superintendent of nurses, everything in and about the place was administered and controlled entirely by a board of men trustees. Finally, it has been my privilege to act as a member of a board of women managers in a hospital administered by both men and women, the former serving in the capacity of trustees, and the women as a board of managers. In addition to this personal experience after watching with keen interest the administration in all sorts and conditions of hospitals, both in this country and abroad, it has become my firm conviction that women are needed in the administration of all such institutions, not just because they are women, or for any Women's Rights" reasons, but because unbiased observation has demonstrated their usefulness, and the influence and part they have taken in establishing and improving hospitals all over the world have become matters of history.

Visitors to a modern well equipped hospital often express surprise when they are told that there are still many people who prefer to struggle through a sickness in the squalor of a tenement house rather than enter the wards where every attention can be paid to them by trained nurses and skilful physicians. Nor do all refuse to accept these advantages from mere blind prejudice, for there is another and a still stronger reason. Despite all the care that is given the patients, there is often something lacking in some of our most noted hospitals which the meanest hovel still offers—an atmosphere of home. "Men may work from sun to sun but woman's work is never done." The former are occupied in the so-called larger fields of the world, but the woman's main occupation is in the home, where she has to deal with men, women and children, at their best and worst, and must be ready to manage intelligently a thousand and one details, if she is to succeed in making a happy home for herself and those around her. As the bread-winner the man must to a large extent devote himself to external matters, and in the matter of home details he becomes accustomed to depend upon the women for carrying out successfully the very many duties with which he is necessarily unfamiliar. It is clear that the same holds good in hospital management. In order to insure the greatest success attainable, the best work of men and women is essential, the former attending to the financial part, and to such affairs as come more strictly within a man's experience, the women looking after the details and the housekeeping part and those affairs belonging to home-life with which they are more conversant. But if we cannot have both then I should without hesitation be in favor of retaining the women and letting the men go, for women have proven themselves to be no mean financiers or planners, where the whole responsibility has rested upon them, and from the standpoint of careful administration and economy they are undoubtedly far ahead of men trustees. One prominent example of which I can speak with knowledge is that of the Illinois Training School for Nurses, Chicago, organized by a few women for the purpose of bringing relief to the city's sick poor by introducing women nurses into the wards of the city and county hospital. This organization has made for itself a name as being the largest school in the country; it provides for the nursing in two of the largest hospitals, and has steadily increased its plant as the need arose.

Moreover, it has not only kept itself free from indebtedness and is practically self-supporting, but for years has been able to make to the public an annual contribution of the income derived from a gift of $50,000, which has been set apart as a special fund and is utilized in supplementing the remuneration of competent trained nurses, who by this means are enabled to take care of the patients of moderate income at reduced charges.

The pupil nurses are well cared for and the school affords an object lesson, teaching the people the duty of providing healthful surroundings for those who care for the sick, and who are sent out to teach by individual example all the possibilities of prophylactic hygienic measures. All this has been accomplished by a board of twenty-four women, and I think we may be well proud of the fact that the duties of superintendent have for years been efficiently carried out by Miss McIsaac, our honorable president.

But it may be asked: Do not the hospital nurses as women represent the home element in these institutions? They undoubtedly do, but it must be remembered that their supervision is restricted chiefly to the wards, and the superintendent is usually the only nurse who has access to all parts of the hospital. If she combines the position of matron with that of superintendent of nurses, she has undoubtedly greater opportunities, but the matron is clever indeed who

in herself possesses all the experience and wisdom
needed to cope with all the details of the various departments as thoroughly, carefully, economically and
perfectly as they should be managed. Besides why
tax and over-work one woman when by a little management and system she may be assisted or relieved
of an unnecessary amount of detail by the willing
co-operation of a number of other women? I have
heard it stated by superintendents on various occasions that these ladies make more work and trouble
than they save. But when this is the case, is it not
possible that the fault lies more with the superintendent than with the board of managers? Naturally the latter cannot expect to know all the ins and
outs of hospital life, but with proper organization
and especially with co-operation on the part of the
superintendent of nurses they grasp the situation in
a surprisingly short time, and hardly ever fail to contribute many good and practical suggestions concerned not only with their own particular duties but
with the good of the whole institution.

But for the accomplishment of the greatest possible
good there are three requisites: (1) a properly selected board of managers; (2) proper organization
and strictly defined duties; and (3) hearty co-operation on the part of the superintendent of nurses. Of
these three the last is the most essential, since a house
divided against itself must inevitably fall, whereas

a united body of workers, even though they may be of no extraordinary individual ability, can accomplish much. The same mind should dwell in all who have anything to do with the hospital, and its best interest and greatest good should always be paramount to private likes and dislikes. The desire to have the opinions of single individuals prevail should always be repressed, and each should determine to take a broad point of view, and accept cheerfully and carry out faithfully any well considered decision of the majority.

In the formation of a board of women managers many things have to be taken into consideration, and it is quite possible that the superintendent of nurses may not always be able to appreciate the various interests to be consulted, so that in some instances it may puzzle her to know why certain women are chosen as members of such a board. The reason governing the selection may vary according to the sources from which the institution is supported. Some hospitals, as we know, are carried on by religious denominations; others are richly endowed by private bequests; in the case of the municipal hospital the cost is provided for out of the city treasury, while others depend for support solely upon public contributions. To this last class belong the greater number. At the same time no matter how securely endowed, or how independent a hospital may be of its public, it is always well to have a number of people in the community who take a personal interest in it, and who are jealous of its good name, who will stand loyally by it if it is unjustly criticised, who will use their influence to make friends for it, and who will see to it that it remains worthy of the favor and confidence of all who may seek its shelter and aid. In these respects the assistance of woman is far-reaching. Again, the active co-operation of well-known women, whose names stand for integrity and what is best in the community, at once lifts any institution with which their names are associated above reproach, and strengthens the hands of the officials in their endeavors at every turn. Moreover, in order that the benefits of the hospital may be made as far-reaching as possible, it is well to have among its supporters those who can serve it not only philanthropically, but also financially, and who can influence others to give. Thus the society woman, the woman who is known for her indefatigable good work, the practical economical housekeeper and the business woman can all find a fitting place on hospital boards.

A proper selection having been made, thorough organization is of vital importance. Each member should be chosen for a definite reason, and her sphere of usefulness having been once recognized, her duties, privileges and restrictions should be defined. Thus a board divided into suitable committees, with an executive committee composed of the heads of these various committees, may be useful in many ways, and will represent and forward all the various interests connected with the institution, of which I need not speak in detail here. Perhaps, however, I may be pardoned for pointing out a few ways in which women members of the board can supplement the work of caring for the sick. For want of time and for absorption in the strictly practical part of their work nurses are apt to forget that there are other factors besires medicines and the routine nursing that act as tonics and aids to the restoration of health, and that convalescence will inevitably be retarded should the patient fall into an indifferent listless attitude of mind. What brightens up the sick more than the sight of a new face, a few fresh flowers, a bright entertaining story or the magazine pictures, a quiet game of some sort, or perhaps some light work for the fingers? All of such things can be supplied by the ward visitor provided the nurses will co-operate far enough to keep her in touch with the patient's needs. Such helps are sources of real economy and great good, for they undoubtedly hasten convalescence so that places are sooner open for others who need the care more. Again, a practical, far-seeing superintendent, who is in hearty accord with her committee on hospital and household supplies, can hold their interest to such an extent that many items will be provided, with a consequent distinct saving to the hospital finances. Again, the individual nurse will find it of great advantage to her when she leaves the hospital to have a certain number of women in the community who are conversant with her ability and her ambitions to further district nursing, visiting nursing or whatever form her future work may take.

In the brief time allotted I have given but imperfectly a few of the many reasons why women are in place on hospital boards, and I beg to close by repeating that it lies in the power of the superintendent of nurses, if she be a capable, experienced executive officer, to utilize these extraneous aids in order to develop more and more the good work done by such boards. Our hospitals of to-day, although far ahead of those of twenty years ago, in some respects still lack the full measure of the home atmosphere that makes patients forget they are within the walls of an institution, and which can only exist where the presence of woman and her aid is appreciated and utilized to the utmost extent possible.

XIII

THE QUALITY OF THOROUGHNESS
IN NURSES' WORK.

THE QUALITY OF THOROUGHNESS IN
NURSES' WORK.*

A LITTLE over thirteen years ago it was my privilege to greet for the first time a Baltimore audience and to become for a few years a resident of Baltimore City. And, like all others who have once lived within her borders or who have been in any way a part of the Johns Hopkins Hospital or University, I have always been eager to seize any opportunity that might afford itself of revisiting the place that has been endeared to me by work and association. So when Dr. Hurd did me the honor to ask me to address the graduates of to-day, the pleasant anticipation of finding myself once more surrounded by Johns Hopkins nurses, past, present and future, and of being again in touch with Baltimore, was not to be withstood. I am only too well aware of the fact that the retrospect and forecast I may hold before you to-day may not contain the full measure of inspiration and wise counsel that you may have hoped for, nor delight you with the happy phrasing that might have been offered you by many others who would gladly have accepted the honor of addressing

---

* Johns Hopkins Hospital, 1903.

you in my place; nevertheless I feel assured that no one could be found who is more profoundly interested than myself in your individual interests and work or who could draw more closely to you in those mutual professional ties and common interests into which you are about to enter.

At that first gathering the Johns Hopkins nurse was conspicuous by her absence. She was still in the future, her place was still to be made in the hospital and household; her history page was still·fair and unwritten. But two years later the first class of graduates stood, where you now stand, prepared to leave their hospital and to go forth to form a new factor in the life of this city, to become part of it for better or worse; and each year since a fresh class has been added to the first until to-day our alumnæ form a goodly host. How they have sped, we of the household, who have watched their individual lives anxiously, know full well. The Johns Hopkins nurse has not only become a familiar presence in many homes both of the needy and of the well-to-do of this city, but to various positions in other cities and countries she has also carried the well-known name of her hospital and school, doing both, we trust, honor and credit.

For the graduate of to-day that first class must need have a special interest, for early in its formation there came into its ranks one who was destined to become, a few years later, the chief executive of your school. From probationer to junior, from grade to grade, she worked her way up until there was no form of nursing within her reach she had not done, no nursing position the hospital had to offer she had not held. Thus year by year she went on with indomitable perseverance, unconsciously training mind and hands, so that when the time came there was no need for the hospital authorities to look beyond their own graduates for a principal for their school for nurses, since they had readily to hand one who was in every way capable of assuming a position of responsibility and trust equalled by few and excelled by none open to members of your profession. And it should be a matter of no small pride and pleasure to all Johns Hopkins nurses that with the exception of the first few years they have held within their own hands the welfare of the nursing department of their own hospital, and at the same time have contributed superintendents for similar positions to other hospitals in a greater proportion for the length of years it has been in existence than perhaps any other school in the country.

But if I recall these facts as affording a sufficient proof of the standard that your school has maintained; if I tell you that the eyes of the hospital world are ever watching with keen interest the progress made by this school, and that the superintendent of your school is an authority on nursing affairs, it is not that you may be puffed up or satisfied with yourselves, but rather realize the burden of the responsibility laid upon you, and that when you have done your best you may say with all humility, "We are unprofitable servants, we have done that which it was our duty to do," and strive to make the future stand for better work than the past.

There is perhaps no other outside of Miss Nutting's immediate co-workers who can be so well aware as myself of the steady progress made by this school; while carrying on its every-day work, she has lost no opportunity for its advancement and betterment, and leaving unmentioned for the moment the many minor but important changes and improvements she has made, it is a great satisfaction to feel that she should have been among the first to inaugurate successfully the three years' course of study, with an eight hours daily system of practical work, which marks one of the greatest advances in training school methods. Her last great achievement has been the establishment of a preliminary course of instruction for probationers, the great need for which has given me a subject ready to hand—a subject that one could readily discourse upon under many and various titles, but to-day permit me to speak of it in its relation to "The Quality of Thoroughness in Nurses' Work."

That there is a deep and widespread dissatisfaction felt at the lack of thoroughness in much of the work to-day and that this deficiency is confined to no particular class of workers, and to no particular degree of service, we are all aware. Nevertheless, although few of us escape the discomfort and annoyance attending upon it in some shape or form, at one time to another, we find ourselves still able to endure it with a certain amount of patience and equanimity, so long as it partakes of the impersonal. But once let it become personal in character, once let it enter the privacy of the home, and we are keenly sensitive and alive to defects in work of any kind and give expression to our feelings and opinions in no uncertain tones. But what worker is brought into more personal and intimate relationship with those with whom she has to deal than the trained nurse? All of us have heard a portion of the public sentimentalize and idealize the nurse with such fulsome flattery that we have sometimes prayed that we might be saved from our friends. On the other hand, we hear daily criticisms upon her many short-comings, and so often are these latter sounded in the ears of the medical practitioner, whose co-worker she is, that he is impelled to look for some favorable opportunity to appease his patients by laying all sorts of injunctions upon the nurse's manners and morals and finds it when making the annual address to the graduating class. And despite the fact that these recommendations have been made, almost without exception, in the kindliest spirit, how often have we, who have had much to do with the making of nurses, been deeply embarrassed that such advice should be deemed necessary, inasmuch as we have felt that if such faults lay wholly and entirely within the guild of nurses we must in common honesty refrain from adding one more member to the list. Graduates of the Johns Hopkins have been favored beyond their kind in having in years gone-by listened in most part to addresses that were an inspiration to better deeds and higher ideals in beginning their professional career. Although you too have been besought upon one or two notable occasions to enter upon your duties in the full consciousness of guilt of such sins and frailties that if you possessed them, and had not battled against them and overcome them long before reaching graduation day, the address of warning would have availed you but little. Do not let me be misunderstood. I am not saying that nurses are perfect. What I wish to point out is that it is more than possible that the glaring imperfections of the trained nurse—and she has many—are not in the main attributable to any lack of training in her profession but are shared by her with her fellows in other walks of life and are the result of inperfect education—and here I use the word education in the broadest sense of the term. In other words inefficiency, superficiality and lack of thoroughness belong not to the graduate nurse alone but are the common property of the modern woman and belong to the average American household.

In the statement that there is a sad lack of thoroughness in the average woman of to-day, I need only refer to training school statistics to bear me out. From one school, in twelve months 1,200 letters of information are sent out and some 175 formal applications are received. Furthermore, from this number only 50 candidates are selected, and nevertheless from this restricted number of women chosen, at least 8 or 10 are dropped generally for inefficiency and lack of education. If then only 40 women, out of a total of 175 applicants, are considered worthy of admission to the school, what is the probable standard of education among the other 135? not to mention the many women who do not make formal application because refusal is certain. Surely the superintendents of training schools are justified in feeling that the unthinking part of the public would have them ''make bricks without straw.''

But the fact that the qualifications of these selected few are not, and never have been, considered by superintendents of training schools of the first order for the making of nurses is now being proved rather by deeds than by words, and this dissatisfaction has found its expression in the establishment of a preliminary course of training, which is being tried in varying degrees in schools of this country and Great Britain and which has been put on a more thorough and comprehensive basis in the Johns Hopkins than elsewhere. This extra course has been made compulsory, before a woman can begin her technical training in nursing, in the hope of overcoming to some extent a very general ignorance and helplessness in a branch of knowledge that for century upon century has been supposed to be woman's chief stronghold—that of household economics. As Miss Nutting has said, "In pursuance of the belief that it is essential for the nurses to have a wide and thorough acquaintance with the subjects of foods and dietetics and a full knowledge of the work of the household, with careful training in its various branches a comparatively large portion of time is devoted to this subject;" and in addition to this special course in Household Economics, some training schools are even advocating and arranging for a course in general literature and in practice in reading aloud, all subjects outside of the direct work of teaching nursing. No doubt many of you might think that the above statement cannot apply to all classes of women, but as a matter of fact actual experience has amply proved that the woman of wealth, the well-to-do woman, and the college student, are equally deficient in manual dexterity so essential to good nursing, and are as ignorant of the underlying principles of household affairs as is the woman who has never had an opportunity to develop her mental powers and has labored all her days with her hands. It can be scarcely appreciated how deficient women are in the practical knowledge of the affairs of the house, until one is brought face to face with such ignorance in some such place as a training school for nurses, where it becomes one of the fundamental requirements. As an example, I have had instructors tell me that not one woman in ten upon first entering the diet school knows how to make a cup of tea properly, few could break an egg deftly enough to separate the yolk from the white, while the qualities of accuracy, precision and a fine finish are invariably absent. The woman who would be a success as a nurse or in fact in anything, who would possess the quality of thoroughness in its fullest sense, no matter what kind of work she undertakes, needs the combined qualities of a trained mind, capable hands and body—and all must be dominated by the soul. Certainly no form of education can make for thoroughness or can fully fit for the business of life that does not recognize an equal training in this great trinity—mind, body and soul.

But when and where should a woman receive such a preparation? Surely not during a six months' preliminary course in a training school for nurses, but rather during the sixteen years preceding the time she is of age to take up the work she intends to make the chief occupation of her life. To quote the words of another, "The hospital is the place *par excellence* to teach the art of nursing and to practise the science, but it is not the best place or even a good place to teach the accessories. Moreover, in assuming the burden of this higher education we are unwisely making ourselves responsible for all the defects and deficiencies in the training of nurses and bearing the criticism against the profession, aimed for the most part not against her nursing education but the accessories." If then this education is to begin with our childhood, where and how should it be given? Naturally in the school and at home. But as Miss Nutting has said, "Were it possible to place the requirements of admission at such a point as would insure in our pupils a definite knowledge of certain prescribed subjects before entrance to the schools of nursing, it is manifest that our work of education might be greatly facilitated." That such a course under present conditions is not practicable is only too evident. Any scheme for such preparatory instruction should include, first a thorough practical training in the care of the household and a knowledge of the properties of foods. Now at present there exists no school of instruction where a candidate could go to prepare herself fitly in these subjects for entrance to the hospital school for nursing. To be sure the Drexel Institute in Philadelphia, the Pratt Institute in Brooklyn, the School of House-keeping in Boston and some others, cover the ground of the domestic sciences admirably, and upon them we draw for our instructors in these branches. But the instruction in these institutions is largely occupied with the subject of foods and cookery, important essentials indeed, but which do not include all that is meant when we say that a pupil should have a knowledge of house-keeping before entering the hospital wards for her training as a nurse. Unfortunately this practical handling of the things and affairs of the home is taught in no schools and in but few homes at the present day,'' and, as Spencer has said, ''That which our school course leaves almost entirely out, we thus find to be that which most nearly concerns the business of life.''

The subject of the home in relation to the question of a three-fold education has of late years been well studied by well qualified investigators who have pointed out clearly and emphatically the shortcomings of the persent day in this connection and have sought for and recommended various remedies through the application of which we may hope to arrive at a better state of affairs; but up to the present time the ground has hardly been broken and no great general advance has been made. Specialized efforts, such as these preliminary courses for student nurses, have already accomplished something directly and indirectly and are doing an immense amount of good, inasmuch as they have emphasized the necessity for similar education in all forms of work.

Thoroughness in any form of education must have its roots deep laid in the home, and we women have much to do with it there, and are answerable in a great measure for the present inefficiency, ignorance, indifference and waste. For the souls of the little children are ours to begin with, "Marvellous delicate and tender things," says Olive Schriner, "and keep forever the shadow that first falls upon them, that is the mother's or at best a woman's." The world requires not more children, but a better quality, not the waste products of human life that so many are to-day. But at the present there seems to be but little hope for that ideal education for the child in whom lies the world's welfare, for the home is one of the few institutions left that still keep the drawbridge up and refuse to let progress and improvement enter within their gates. The individual still regards his home as his castle, in its most conservative sense, and still clings to old traditions, old systems and time-honored cook-books, and refuses to come into line and be guided by association and combination, by economic laws and principles, and by the specialization of labor in its true sense which makes for thoroughness as no other way can.

But women cannot be held entirely responsible for

the increasing difficult conditions in the household, and for the wholesale lack of thoroughness within and without. Progress in many forms has taken out of it a great variety of work that was once done in the household by women and the time formerly spent in these various duties has not been fully accounted for in other forms of activities. How long will it still be assumed about house-keepers, as it formerly was about nurses, that they are born and not made and that the only essential required is to be a woman; that a taste and knowledge for all things domestic is hers by divine right, that she intuitively knows all about the care and bringing up of children, the laws of health, hygiene, sanitation, foods and their preparation, suitable clothing and furnishings. And yet such a groundless assumption leaves her at the mercy of two very unstable teachers, Instinct and Experience, the former sometimes lacking, and the latter at all times to be acquired at a great cost. So at the present moment we have the spectacle of each household trying to be a training school unto itself in domestic affairs, wasting the time of both mistress and maid in vainly trying to teach and to do things without any adequate knowledge of underlying principles, busy making patients for the doctor and nurse by jeopardizing the health of families by their woeful ignorance, and later themselves falling by the wayside a prey to worry and worn-out nerves.

Nor are these the least of the woes that befall the modern household through its want of proper organization, its oldtime methods and its modern dangers. The rapid accumulation of great wealth and its consequent tendency to luxurious forms of living and ease have brought us very near to that point in the order of social change when a large class of women are in danger of becoming useless supernumeraries without an excuse for existing and a menace to the nation. The average man of the day devotes his energies early and late in the making of money, economizing labor at all points to compass his purpose, only to end in pouring his wealth into the hands of a wife or children who expend it in such profusion and lavishness of ignorance, as has made Americans stand for greater extravagance than perhaps any other civilized people.

Even a superficial consideration of the question then will readily show that the inefficiency of the trained nurse can justly be placed only where it belongs—in the lack of proper early education; and while the preliminary course of instruction for other reasons is excellent and will probably always exist, it is to be hoped that it will not always be necessary to devote so large a portion of the time to Household Economics. Any adequate remedy for the present state of affairs can only come through a true education of our women. They must be trained, disci-

plined to bear their due share of the work needful for
the helping of the nation; they must be taught that
the true value of money lies not in the luxury it
may heap about them, but in the opportunities it
affords, and that the true joy of living can only be
found in congenial work. It would be well if all appreciated the fact that the existing or faulty order
must inevitably continue until our women of wealth,
refinement and intellectual attainments combine their
talents, leisure and intelligence to bring the home into its proper place in the economic and scientific world
by the readjustment of household work and by creat-
ing the desire and the demand that our sons and
daughters, children of all ranks and grades, should
be given a proper education; that from the beginning
there shall go hand in hand the teaching of their
numberless faculties that shall make for a practical
and proper appreciation of the principles of art, education and labor and the joy to be found in each.
For then and then only can they understand what
life means and know how to live. Moreover, the preparation must be such an one as shall be a fitting preliminary training for their future occupation in life,
whether it be that of the trained nurse, the physician,
the house-keeper, statesman, artist or artisan; each
one whether man or woman, being prepared to fill
their chosen niche, happy in having found it and not,
as now too often happens, being forced into occupa-

tions for which they often have neither the heart, head nor hand.

Upon both men and women are we dependent for the first steps that shall establish and thoroughly equip professional schools for the investigation of all subjects pertaining to the household, and that shall offer suitable inducements only to such persons as have the proper attainments for carrying on such studies, after which we may look for the establishment of technical schools for children, embracing all branches of work that in any manner touch the home. These schools should cover the country like a network, as do the public schools, and should co-operate with them; they too should have the authority of the law behind them for which the rank and the file of the people have due respect. In such schools should the trained nurse find her proper place. With her more intimate knowledge of disease and its causes and the dangers that menace health, she is well fitted to be the teacher of home sanitation, hygiene, the personal laws of health, the true meaning of cleanliness and the prevention of disease. Despite the fact that bacteriologists are every day throwing more light upon the causes of disease, and each city is equipped with its health officer, hospitals are still being multiplied in the land, the supply of trained nurses is not equal to the demand, and our wards are just as full of typhoid fever patients as of yore. These facts must sometimes make us pause to question if we are not spending our labor and strength for that which profiteth not. But thus it must be until the public at large and as individuals have acquired a practical intelligent appreciation of the above subjects and of the duties of individuals and communities in the prevention of disease.

We need two orders of trained nurses, the new order of the co-operating health nurse with the old order for the sick, who must ever be with us. The appointment of a staff of trained nurses to the schools of New York by the Health Commission for the purpose of continuing the work in the public schools is the beginning of this new order, and is a hopeful sign of the times.

Graduates of to-day, we who are already of the guild greet you heartily and give you cordial welcome to your place among us. In your future work we see much of hope and promise. When you have grown a little older and have had a more varied experience, you will realize that the mere care of the patient is the least part of your work compared with what you can and ought to do towards making the conditions that cause pain and sickness and all manner of suffering less possible.

In the last issue of *The American Journal of Nursing,* Miss Dock says: "After one has worked for a time in healing wounds which should never have been inflicted, tending illness which should never have developed, sending patients to hospitals who need not have gone if their homes were habitable, bringing charitable aid to persons who would not have needed charity if health had not been ruined by unwholesome conditions, one loses heart and longs for preventive work, constructive work—something that will make it less easy for so many illnesses and accidents to occur, that will help to bring better homes and workshops, better conditions of life and labor." And this expressed longing finds its echo in the heart of each of us who have learned by experience that the faithful nursing of the patient, the splendid work done in so many forms of philanthropy and the efforts of religion do not reach the root of the matter. In your professional life you have learned that we may dress and nurse a wound ever so carefully, but that all your work represents time and energy expended in vain, that a breakdown of the wound is inevitable, did not the surgeon first clean and scrape away all the diseased tissues, reaching deep down into the fresh healthy part until no germ of disease was left to impair the growth of new, healthy flesh. And so it is with our work in caring for humanity in other ways —we are but staying a worse condition perhaps, but not removing the cause if we rest satisfied with mere treatment and do not direct our best energies towards prevention.

You are, therefore, to be congratulated in your choice of work, you are entering a field of labor that is ever widening and where each can make for herself a definite place in rendering such ideals of education, as I have but haltingly tried to show you today, practical facts. More especially are you to be congratulated in your choice of a school where the standard of excellence desired for its graduates is so clearly set forth, and where there is placed within the reach of pupils the possibility of that quality of thoroughness that is the great need and demand of the day.

XIV

THE AFFILLIATION OF TRAINING SCHOOLS FOR EDUCATIONAL PURPOSES.

THE AFFILIATION OF TRAINING SCHOOLS FOR EDUCATIONAL PURPOSES.*

O N first thought it might seem more fitting that the subject of this paper should be presented before the Society of Superintendents of Training Schools, inasmuch as the carrying out of such a scheme must have a direct bearing upon the work of the individual superintendents and upon the object of that society. On the other hand, a federation meeting should be an advantageous ground upon ·which to array affiliation forces, since a federation already accomplished not only affords a stimulus towards a further extension of the idea along lines which, although differing in kind and degree, are fundamentally similar, but also supplies experience which may be utilized in determining how this extension may be brought about.

"It is with a little hesitation that I approach a discussion of the affiliation of training schools for nurses, knowing that the plan is fraught with many difficulties that can only be met through the united

---

* Federation of Nurses Convention, Washington, 1905.

deliberations and with the common consent of such bodies as are most nearly concerned.

"The past fifteen years have found us as individuals and as associations busy over improvements in nursing conditions and the education of the nurse. On the whole, it may be said that the progress made has been steady and encouraging, but considering that we had practically a fresh, uncultivated field in which to work, it would be little to our credit as interested, intelligent workers were we not able to point to marked improvements over our first tentative beginnings. Of course, in great undertakings fifteen years is a very small space of time, and on account of the youth of the movement our efforts have necessarily partaken largely of the experimental. Nevertheless, we may congratulate ourselves that this experimental stage has now lasted long enough to justify us in drawing a certain number of definite conclusions as to the value of the methods so far employed. Moreover, now that we are able to see just where we stand in respect to educational matters we can better realize how present conditions may be affected by the affiliation proposition.

"It is hardly necessary to mention in detail all the work we have accomplished through mutual and associated effort. Fortunately, I think we can be reasonably certain that little or no time has been entirely lost; that so far as we have gone there is not much to regret or to wish undone, and that our efforts thus far have resulted in a great deal of general good. But recognizing the fact that all our experimental work has been a necessary preparation for development on more original and broader lines in the future, it may be well at the present time to devote a few moments to the consideration of such steps as have had a direct bearing upon the educational advancement of the members of the nursing profession.

"From the first those of us who have been intimately associated with the organization and development of nursing have recognized that very difficult and serious problems had to be met and solved if we would have nursing organization stand for something more than mere numbers,—quantity without quality, —and if we nurses were finally to qualify ourselves in deed as well as in word to enter into the full privileges afforded to members of a profession. Such privileges should presuppose certain requirements, which, broadly speaking, are three in number: first, there must be a definite educational standard; secondly, a proper professional spirit; thirdly, recognition by the public of this professional standard. To provide means for the satisfaction of these requirements has been the aim of our two great associations of nurses. From the first the Society of Superintendents has had as its primary object the educational advancement of nursing and the development of a fixed standard of education that should be common to all schools and to all nurses. On the other hand, the Associated Alumnæ, while working for the general uplifting of the nurse and her work, has sought for proper protection by the law and recognition by the public. The demand to some extent for improved educational conditions for training schools has been the outcome of the putting into practice of some of the nurses' own ideals whereby the medical profession has been taught to expect more and better things of the nurse Again, as we all know, the advancement in medicine and surgery calls for a greater degree of skill, knowledge, and integrity on the part of the nurse. And, lastly, we have come to recognize that no public recognition could very well be asked for unless we had some sort of an educational standard upon which to base our claims. The first general steps were comparatively simple. A minimum of two years as a standard time for the education of the student nurse was already in existence, although there were some exceptions to the rule. The division of this period into junior and senior work with schedules of classes, lectures, and demonstrations in certain subjects appropriate to each year was no great feat, although were we to-day to examine carefully into the arrangement of such schedules, into the subjects taught and the ground covered in each, and into the methods employed, we should find a great diversity, more modifications by far than was justifiable or necessary to meet the individual needs of each hospital. Next, the practice of sending the student nurse out to do nursing in private families during her time of training was by a strenuous effort on the part of both associations largely done away with, thus enabling the student to profit by systematic instruction in the hospital during the full term of two years.

"Nevertheless, we still find it cropping up insidiously under the protection of the additional third year and under the guise of an educational feature.

"But the first change of real note was the lengthening of the term of training from two to three years, until the latter period has in this country become the time generally adopted, although we cannot say it has become the universal standard, since some schools still offer courses ranging from two to two and a half years, while others have forged ahead and are requiring three and a half to four years. Nor can we say that this increase in the duration of the training has always been very advantageous from a purely educational standpoint; for it is obvious to all that while the added year of experience is of undoubted value to the student, the hospital of the two reaps the greater benefit, particularly when the nurse's hours on duty have not been shortened. Many hospitals have adopted with readiness the third year, but only here and there, in very few schools indeed, have the hours in the wards been reduced to even eight practical hours of work. To add on a whole year to the course of training and claim that it is for educational improvement is manifestly a delusion unless a fair proportion of the extra time is devoted to study alone. And we all know that the capacity for mental effort in the average person counts for little after nine or ten hours of ordinary physical work, which is entirely free from the additional nervous strain attendant upon nursing. In respect to hours on duty, therefore, we are still far from a generally accepted educational standard.

"Again, it has been conceded that the old-time method of giving a monthly allowance to each pupil was to be deplored on the principle that it lessened the educational value of the instruction and that it was far better to give an education commensurate with the services rendered. As a result, the monthly allowance is gradually being done away with—somewhat slowly, in fact, for the system of offering a small monthly compensation or a fixed sum at the end of the term of training is still practised in some schools which, it may be, do not feel sufficient confidence in the educational advantages they offer to lessen their chances for drawing the required number of desirable candidates by cutting off so powerful an inducement as this undoubtedly is to many good women. On the other hand, some few schools have gone even beyond the non-payment system and are requiring fixed entrance fees, ranging from twenty-five dollars to fifty dollars and one hundred dollars. In this respect, then, we are again far from a common standard.

''The subject of dietetics has received more and more attention until a practical and theoretical course of instruction in this branch of nursing is now regarded as necessary and is given in about every school. But too often we find the course is not arranged primarily from an educational standpoint, but rather is looked upon as a valuable asset in the economics of the hospital. And where shall we find any two schools that agree as to how the subject should be taught and how much time shall be devoted to it? All are so varied that no possible standard could be arrived at.

''A fresh impetus has been given to this particular branch of nursing and to that of household economics in relation to nursing by the reorganization and extension of that part of the teaching into a preliminary course of training, but in the plan of reorganization and systematization of the teaching we again find a great lack of uniformity. Preliminary courses at present range from three to four and six months, and the methods employed in the selection of subjects and in the manner of teaching them vary widely. Moreover, if the establishment of a preliminary course means that the hospital has an additional class to house and keep for from four to six months before the members enter the wards the added expense will certainly preclude the general adoption of a most valuable arrangement.

"Nor have we even an approximate standard of qualifications for the acceptance or rejection of applicants or for the dismissal of delinquent students; for a woman who may be regarded by one superintendent as an unfit probationer and is therefore refused, or a pupil who has been dismissed for reasonable cause, may promptly be accepted by another superintendent and will ultimately be allowed to graduate. Finally the Teachers' Course in Hospital Economics has been sufficiently long in existence to prove to us that, while excellent in its way so far as it goes, it can never be the ultimate means of regulating the standard of education for nursing.

"These represent some of the principal measures that have had more or less of a trial and are familiar to most of us, as they have all been subjects for papers and discussions before the Superintendents' Society for some twelve years. And I would ask you to note the fact that whereas in almost every instance some attempt at accepting the whole or some part of some suggested improvement in methods has been made by individual schools, curiously enough in no single case has the society ever taken concentrated action, or pledged itself to the general adoption of any one form of improvement or to accept any standard so far proposed, feeling, no doubt, that such a measure would be impracticable. This means that, so far as the society is concerned, although through its efforts the general improvement has been amazing, we are as far from a generally accepted standard of education as we were in the beginning, so that we must perforce conclude under *present conditions* we can expect little, if any, more in this direction than we have already accomplished.

"The actual establishment of anything approaching a standard has been brought about by the nurses as a body through their Associated Alumnæ. With the desire for legal protection and for some sort of legal recognition by the public there came at once the recognition of the imperative necessity for establishing something approaching to a common standard of education for all nurses who might seek to qualify for State registration. It became, therefore, one of the first duties of the Boards of Examiners in those States in which State registration has been legalized to prepare a standard of education for each particular State. Here at once great difficulties were encountered, and through the disability of graduates of certain schools in these States to qualify we are now brought face to face with the problem which must be solved in order to save disruption and confusion. How, then, shall we proceed to bring such schools into line for the purpose of State registration? The natural solution would seem to be through the affiliation of the various schools for educational purposes.

"But there are reasons other than these concerned with State registration which render it important that some such plan should be adopted. In the first place, in this country, at least, State registration cannot set a national standard, inasmuch as the laws governing each State differ in many respects. Furthermore, although the standard set in certain States may be all that can be reasonably desired under present conditions, there is always the danger that amendments injurious to such a standard may be introduced and that in others it may be set unreasonably low to begin with. Moreover, how can any State require all its training schools for nurses to come up to a given standard when not all of the hospitals in which schools exist are or ever can be general hospitals? Under present conditions, then, there will always remain some which will never be able to comply with the State requirements unless means are afforded them with this end in view. Such means must be first provided before any good standard can reasonably be required, and I am sure that the hospitals which are deficient would gladly avail themselves of increased facilities. When we read of what has been done in 'the best schools' the idea must surely strike us that where the sick are concerned there should be no best schools. Nevertheless, although it stands to reason that various grades of hospitals exist and must continue to exist and that all cannot afford equal opportunities for the education of nurses, it does not necessarily follow that the sick should be less efficiently cared for in one kind of hospital than in the other, provided that the women who wish to become nurses are supplied with equal advantages for rendering themselves competent. Our aim and desire, then, should be to establish a good uniform education for all nurses in every State and in all hospitals. Some system must be elaborated whereby we may obtain this uniform education, and until this is accomplished our sympathies must lie with the hospitals of limited opportunities.

"As a matter of fact, to my knowledge no hospital now exists at present where such a uniform education can be acquired. In matters of general training the large general hospital offers the larger field for experience than could be found in a similar institution of smaller capacity. Of course, the special hospitals do not offer scope enough, but when it comes to a definition of a full general training then it is equally true that the large general hospital must look to other sources for supplying a training in certain branches to round off its course. If, then, we set up as a standard a full general training, we must admit that neither the large nor the small hospital is complete enough to be quite independent, and that for lack of system, proper organization, and affiliation students in every hospital are every day losing valuable practical experience in different branches of nursing. We have given the independent method of carrying on training schools a fair trial, and our results have proved deficient. Each school has gone its own way, apparently indifferent to or careless of the well-being of the whole. Fortunately, however, this 'I am superior and better than my neighbor' attitude has been in a great measure only in the seeming. We know that a very different spirit exists, and that, although not always openly expressed, the hearty desire for the general betterment has a real existence. Hospital authorities and superintendents of training schools have done to the best of their ability, and have utilized approximately to the limit the possibilities of the system under which they have been hampered and under which they have had to work. The main limitation is based upon the fundamental fact that from the educational standpoint the relation of the training school to the hospital has always been an impossible one. With our present system the hospital work has always come first, and the nurses' education has been relegated to a secondary position. The system is responsible for the fact that undesirable candidates are frequently accepted, because the work of the hospital must go on whether the proper standard of nursing is maintained or not, even at the risk of forfeiting the best results for the hospital as well as the highest excellence for the nurse. In this, as in most other instances, superintendents of school have been powerless to do more than they have already done.

"In no instance has a training school for nurses been founded primarily as an educational institution; it has always been regarded as an appendage to a hospital. But until this is changed and schools for nurses are founded for the primary purpose of educating women in nursing—the hospital being utilized as the ground for gaining practical experience—we can scarcely hope for any uniformity among nurses or for the highest grade of work for the hospital or the sick. The best medical schools now stand on this basis and the results are more and more gratifying. How can schools for nurses be established on a similar basis? Even at the present day I believe this end may be largely accomplished by a proper affiliation of the schools which now exist.

"The subject of affiliation is not a new one with us, for the existence of difficult problems connected with the bringing of the small general and specialty hospital into line for educational purposes was recognized years ago. My paper on 'Nursing in Small

General and Specialty Hospitals,' read before the Society of Superintendents in 1897, would seem not to be out of date even at the present, and to a certain extent might still be employed to supplement the present one. In it I explained in detail the need for a general nursing standard and for coöperation of larger with smaller hospitals. Coöperative nursing was tried as early as 1888, when the Illinois Training School of Chicago undertook for a given sum the entire nursing of the Presbyterian Hospital of that city. This arrangement was made with the object of supplying a training for the students of the Illinois Training School in the care of private ward patients, and of doing away with the necessity of sending pupil nurses out to private duty. At the same time it did away with the small training school attached to the Presbyterian Hospital for the reason that the opportunities were limited to certain kinds of nursing and the training was inadequate. This was my first experience in coöperative nursing, but ever since I have been a firm believer in some such plan as the ultimate basis of training for all schools. Since that time more or less coöperative nursing has been attempted. At one time in Milwaukee a central school had under its charge as many as nine hospitals, and within the past three or four years quite a long list of schools could be named that have coöperated, usually with the view of supplementing some branch of training that was lacking. How permanent these later efforts at coöperation may be remains to be seen. Such experiments, however, were always heretofore short lived, and without going accurately into statistics I may say that the majority of these earlier attempts sooner or later ended in disruption. The arrangement made by the Illinois Training School lasted perhaps longer than any other, some fifteen years elapsing before its final withdrawal from its nursing relations with the Presbyterian Hospital. An account of the many causes for the failure of this plan of nursing would be too lengthy to give here and would not be particularly to the point, but one chief impediment to its success and general adoption lies in the difficulty of adapting the methods of one school to those of another without too mch repetition and loss of time and some friction. Were there one generally recognized standard, the same curriculum, and only certain definite teaching required of each school so affiliated, these objections would not hold to the same extent. That coöperative nursing thus far has not proved an unqualified success is not surprising. That any degree of success has been attained is extraordinary for the reason that the plan was not started on the right basis. The added experience of years has taught that the chief obstacle lies in the fact that the necessary stability is lacking in that those most nearly concerned have never been afforded proper representation in the administration of the coöperative plan. The balance of power usually centered in the school that contracted to do all the nursing or to provide a certain branch of training for another hospital. The hospital thus cared for after the financial consideration had been agreed upon had practically no voice in the choice of the methods to be employed in the nursing. With our love for the personal note, it is only natural that each superintendent of nurses and each hospital should wish to have a voice in the arrangements for the education of one's own students and in the administration of so important a department of the hospital as that of nursing.

"Such considerations and others of equal importance must therefore be borne in mind. In endeavoring, then, to arrange for the affiliation of training schools I would advocate the establishment of central institutes in each State offering a comprehensive theoretical and practical training in general nursing. Such institutes would be independent of any particular hospital, but would be organized and administered through a central committee composed of the proper representatives from the hospitals and schools entering into the affiliation. The proper representatives would be chosen from among those most nearly concerned in the welfare of each hospital—namely, the trustees of the hospital, the medical staff, the superintendent of the hospital, and the principal of the training-school. A proper selection of this board is the first essential, for with the best intentions in the world no outside element could fully understand or successfully deal with the particular needs and conditions belonging to the education of nurses. From these several sources a properly balanced committee on training-school affairs should be selected, such committees combined forming the central committee of the central nursing institute. The institute, be it distinctly understood, would have to do not only with preliminary courses in connection with the preparation of candidates, but would be responsible for the entire education in general nursing of accepted candidates. Upon this central committee would devolve the fixing of a standard of general training, the preparation of a general curriculum, the selection of lecturers, instructors, and inspectors, the determination of a plan of rotation from one hospital to another, the definite ground to be covered in each hospital, and the management of the finances of the institute. This central committee would be divided into the necessary sub-committees, among which might be mentioned the Committee on Finance and the committee dealing with the admission of probationers, inasmuch as all applicants to any school in affiliation would be referred to the central institute for acceptance or rejection. Such a committee would naturally be composed of the principals of the affiliated training schools. In order to take in all the hospitals in a large or populous State, the establishment of two or more such institutes might be necessary, but all would be organized on the same basis and all examinations would be held at the same time all over the State. All diplomas would issue from the nursing institute and not from any one hospital.

"Broadly speaking, in arriving at a standard of training it would be necessary to decide upon the requirements for entrance and the length of the preliminary course and of the course of training, and the subjects required to be taught and practised, and the arrangement of the curriculum for the several years. Each central institute would provide a set of regular lectures and a course of instruction. The head of the institute might also under the direction of the central committee act as inspector of the several affiliated training schools. The various hospitals would be arranged into groups in such a way that each group would provide a full course of training. The method of distributing the students to each of such groups would also have to be arranged. The Finance Committee would deal with endowments, scholarships, fees, lectures, and instructors' salaries, the pooling of the expenses, and the like. These and many other matters present problems which are of vital importance, and which must be satisfactorily dealt with before affiliation can attain even a measure of success. In the present paper they cannot be dealt with in detail.

"The advantages of a successful affiliation would be manifold. First and foremost, the establishment of the much to be desired standard could be brought about, and in all forms of hospitals the nursing would be uniform, this uniformity rendering State registration comparatively easy to attain. Moreover, the sick in our hospitals and homes could feel assured of better nursing.˙ The preliminary course would be assured to all students without additional cost to the individual hospital. The arrangement would also tend largely towards economy, since much repetition would be saved and the number of instructors and lecturers would be minimized. Being primarily educational, the course of training would attract a more uniformly desirable class of women. Again, the superintendents of the training schools would be relieved of much clerical work and saved many interruptions. They would individually be relieved of the selection and care of probationers, and would thus be enabled to systematize their time better and to spend more of it in the wards, where their powers of observation, teaching, and influence are of so much practical value.

"The whole aim of the central institute should be towards thoroughness and the production of quality rather than quantity. It should, therefore, in addition to the undergraduate education, provide postgraduate courses in general nursing and a special course in every special form of nursing that is allied with medicine. All such courses must be thorough. Three years should be a sufficient time in which to cover the course in general training, and if a woman is to spend more than three years in learning to be a nurse the extra time, over and above the three prescribed years, should be devoted to optional work and special training in some particular branch of nursing for which a student has shown a particular aptitude. At the present day in the world's work there is a general tendency towards coöperation—towards the formation of trusts if you will—and towards specialization of a high order in all branches. For it stands to reason that after a thorough general groundwork has been laid, the individual who selects a particular branch from natural taste, inclination, and adaptability is bound to carry that branch to a higher degree of excellence and gain better results than is possible when the energy is diffused over a wide field. As in medicine, so in nursing, the specialist is bound to come more and more into evidence, and nursing work must naturally be subdivided. Already we find distinct specialists in our midst—the district nurse, the army nurse, the superintendent of the general hospital and training school, the superintendent of the special hospital—for children, for contagious diseases, for obstetrics, for tuberculosis, for nervous diseases and insanity. Add to these the instructor in dietetics, the sanitary inspector, the school nurse, the masseuse, and we have already a goodly list that need special methods for their proper preparation, other than those that have formed a necessary part of the training in general nursing. But so far as the central institute is concerned, only those subjects that pertain primarily to the nursing of disease should find their place in the general curriculum. The specialties must fall into subdivisions and groups, standing for certain objects. Thus district nursing includes more than the nursing of sick poor; it deals with a branch of social economics in which the nursing itself takes a secondary place, the nurse serving as an instructor in the art of right living and the maintenance of health. Such a specialty, although it requires as a general basis the course in general nursing, calls for a knowledge of certain social conditions that could not possibly be treated properly during the ordinary course of training. Again, as regards the making of superintendents and instructors, only here and there do we meet with a woman who shows the natural executive ability to manage large affairs in a business-like way, or who possesses the faculty of imparting knowledge to others in a clear manner; and only those who can profit by them should have the larger and special opportunities for developing this natural gift.

"Nor is it necessary that provision for every form of teaching should be supplied by the centralized school when by means of affiliation with institutions dealing with other forms of work we can obtain what is particularly needed to supplement our own teaching. For example, for teachers' work a nurse might take a prescribed course in Teachers College, New York, for social work a course in the School of Philanthropy, Boston, or similar institutions.

"Our great trouble has been that seeing all these many fields of usefulness ready for nurses and needing workers, for want of a proper system and classification we have frantically tried to add on a little instruction in each to the list belonging to the general nursing curriculum, with the result that no one of them is dealt with thoroughly, and that the special student is unsatisfied, and the general student has one additional burden to carry. If we are willing to reorganize our training schools on the basis of a general theoretical and practical education that will embrace all hospitals and all subjects pertaining to the care of the sick and rigidly relegate all other subjects to their proper place as specialties to be taken up only by the women who have the natural ability and taste for them, we shall in the course of time reap some very satisfactory results in both the general nursing and the specialties. And to-day no better methods suggest themselves to my mind than those which could be provided through the affiliation of all hospitals for nursing purposes on some such basis as I have endeavored to present to you.''

XV

THE NURSE AS A CITIZEN.

THE NURSE AS A CITIZEN.*

WHENEVER the opportunity comes to me of foregathering with those of my kind it has always seemed well worth the effort to overcome distance and adjust duties for the sake of the pleasure and profit that I gain from such meetings. But in this particular instance, my dear Canadian nurses, your kind invitation touched a still deeper chord, for it came as a call to one who twenty-four years ago was among the first to leave her Canadian home to enter upon what at that time was a comparatively new field of activity for women. Since then most of my work has been done in another country, but to the "native-born" the years and the countries cannot diminish the love for one's own land—"They change the skies above them, but not their hearts that roam" and the opportunities to come back are hailed with joy. And if after all these years of varied experience and contact with nurses and nursing affairs and with the great world of people I can bring back to my younger Canadian sisters anything that may in the slightest degree be suggestive in the advancement of their work; if anything I may be able to tell you will

---

* Toronto Trained Nurses' Club, 1906.

serve to help you, however little, in your chosen work my visit will bring to me a twofold pleasure.

In asking me to speak upon ''The Nurse as a Citizen,'' I take it, you wished me to deal not so much with the older and long accepted formulæ but rather with the newer and ever broadening citizenship that the 20th century is opening up to men and women. For there can be no manner of doubt that forces are at work in the world to-day that are gradually bringing to us a deeper and truer realization of the meaning of life and in a new conception of its significance that must ultimately result in a higher standard of citizenship for all of us. Consciously or unconsciously all of us must be helpers or hinderers in this rapidly spreading movement for the uplifting of mankind, for it finds its expression in many ways and one stumbles upon it in unexpected quarters. Already so many beacon lights from high vantage ground stand to point the way that I feel it were somewhat presumptuous on my part to attempt to direct your thoughts towards any one object. In literature higher standards for mankind have already been dealt with so searchingly and so convincingly as to require the most deep and thoughtful study on our part. In practice this feeling is finding its expression in different ways; philanthropy, associated and individual, is reaching out in many directions, supplying the necessary means for our present needs

and an effective aid in bridging the present with that
future when the world's needs shall be met by other
and better methods than those we must now accept
in the name of charity, correction and philanthropy.
The churches are also keeping pace with the social
movements. Here and there education is being developed upon more pratical lines; labor unions are
the expression of a desire on the part of the masses
for a higher and better condition of social affairs, and
scientific medicine is showing the way to combat disease in some of its most terrible forms. That nurses
in Canada have been touched by the same spirit is
evidenced by your past achievements and can be de-
tected in the selection of subjects for your course of
lectures this winter, it is evident in many ways that
you are drawing together and at some personal and
financial sacrifice are trying to put yourselves in the
way of learning more fully what further share you
may take in advancing the greater good. You have
already discussed the position of the nurse in relation to visiting nursing, in nursing in the home, in
the public schools in the fight against tuberculosis,
and in the roll of inspector of tenement houses. In
what further ways then can nurses qualify for citizenship of the higher order?

But before we can attempt further advancement,
we must be sure we can qualify for the ordinary accepted code in citizenship. In return for the privi-

leges and rights conferred upon each as a member of
a civil society certain obligations are laid upon the
members, which briefly are to be law-abiding, to render allegiance, service and money according to one's
status and means to the country in which one lives.
All good citizens interpret these obligations in a
Christian and liberal sense; churches are built and
supported; hospitals and free libraries are endowed;
cities are beautified at private cost; societies of various sorts are organized for the improvement and benefit of all who reside within a particular city, state
or country. These are a few of the many ways with
which we are all familiar and in which a woman who
later on becomes a nurse has the privilege of par-
ticipating as a good citizen, even before she enters a
training school. Nevertheless it is probable that she
is not made to realize her obligations to any extent,
for thus far little public spirit or service is expected
of a woman in private life, unless it is her will and
pleasure to give it. But when a woman enters a
training school for nurses all this changes, for she at
once becomes an accepted servant of the public, and
what she does and how she does it carries with it far
more weight than her doings in private life—and
more is expected of her. It is, therefore, important
that she faithfully observe at least all the obligations
of citizenship to which she has been accustomed to
conform. Nor are these always so easy of accom-

plishment as it may seem, for many things combine
to make it hard and even irksome for a woman to
continue the even tenor of her life. During her training the absorption in her duties, the effort of acquiring special kinds of knowledge and the extra fatigue
leave little time and energy for extraneous duties, so
that unless habits of system, order and economy in
performing her duties and regulating her time are
well looked after many things are sacrificed, many
good habits may be let go and other undesirable ones
take their places. To begin with, the custom of going
to church is one that may be easily let go. Duties
or fatigue, or both may interfere at first, the older
students may not go, and the force of example is
strong, until finally the staying away becomes a con-
firmed habit and with it goes the obligation to contribute to the support of the church. Thus, when
her three years are up and the woman graduates she
is cut off from a good habit and an obligation of her
private life that made for good citizenship. Again,
during her training a woman is in danger of losing
her sense of appreciation of values. Probably in her
home she may have been made to know the value of
the materials employed and has had to contribute her
share towards care and economy in their use; but in
the hospital she finds herself provided with the necessities and comforts of a home for which she has not to
give any thought; in her work in the wards, food,

linen, light and supplies in plenty are supplied without any exercise of forethought on her part, and are accepted as a matter of course. Hence the sense of responsibility is apt to fall from her and she may fail to realize that she is the steward and dispenser of public benefits, and that according to her use or abuse a larger or smaller number of the sick will be deprived of necessary aid . Thus if she neglects to see her duties in this respect, after graduation when she enters upon private duty the obligations connected with care and economy in the home are forgotten and in this way she is lacking in good citizenship. Had I the time I might mention many other obligations that may be lost sight of in the transition period from private to public life, but these two are perhaps the most important and the ones that would impress the public first. Again, among the unbusiness-like habits are sometimes to be noted in the graduate nurse the lack of the sense of obligation in keeping her appointments, the tardiness in answering a call to a patient at once after she has reported herself as ready to do so; neglect to notify her directory, her professional societies and her Nursing Journal of her change of address and many other little negligences, they might be called, but in reality serious sins of omission. Women in private life are notorious for a lack of business habits and of a sense of responsibility that calls for punctuality in keeping engagements, but these offences are condoned or even smiled at. The nurse, however, must make up her mind from the very beginning that in the public life which she has assumed observance of all the responsibilities becomes a cardinal principle and that if she fails in these ordinary obligations of private and professional life, the public can very justly question her capacity for performing the more serious duties involved in her special work. Owing to neglect in this respect our standards and influence are at times materially lessened and all suffer for the faults of a few. Nor can we possibly enter upon higher development unless we first practice these fundamental principles. Graduates as a body then, have to meet their obligations as private citizens which existed before and in addition those that they assume when they become members of a profession that is for the use of the public, for upon this professional body is laid the obligation of rendering to the public service of the highest order. While still in the hospital it may seem to the woman in training that to be a graduate from a good school and hospital will always carry with it a sufficient recommendation, and that only from these standards will she be judged. But after graduating she finds that quite the reverse obtains and that the public regards her merely as a trained nurse and pays little heed to the particular hospital or school, and that she will have to suffer at least for her own shortcoming if not for those of others as well. She also finds that school standards and educational advantages vary greatly, and that what really constitutes a qualified graduate nurse is a question that has not yet found its solution. Happily in the United States we have already recognized our deficiencies, as is evidenced by the establishment of our Alumnæ Associations, our local and State Associations, our National Association, our Superintendents' Society and our Nursing Journals. One chief outcome of all this association work, has been as you know, the work towards State Registration for Nurses, and these efforts have brought us face to face with the fact that educationally we have no recognized standard, and that it has been impossible to fix upon an even moderately high standard for which the majority of graduates could qualify without special preparation, for the reason that they had graduated from schools connected with hospitals that did not furnish opportunities for practical nursing and teaching in many of the branches requisite for the thorough training of a nurse. As it is impossible for the average hospital to embrace the care of all forms of diseases, the natural solution to the problem would seem to lie in the affiliation of hospitals and training schools for educational purposes—and on this basis we are just now trying to reach a standard.

So far have we in the United States met one of our

higher obligations of citizenship—to render a genuinely efficient nursing service to the public—that we have much hard work ahead of us before we actually succeed we all realize.

In Canada nurses have the same difficulties to face only in a lesser degree and under infinitely more favorable circumstances. Whereas, we must need establish registration state by state and even then with vastly varying standards, you have but to make your efforts towards a national issue with one standard for all provinces. You have therefore every incentive to make your requirements such as must finally give to Canada a uniformly high grade of nurse and of nursing service. And as we know that the affiliation of hospitals and schools must go hand in hand with registration to provide the full requirements of practical training, I would beg of you to direct your efforts towards the establishment of central provincial schools which shall be independent of any particular hospital, but which shall equally belong to and be controlled by all affiliated hospitals, thus doing away with the present system of schools as appendages to hospitals, and placing them on a purely educational basis from which the same efficient nursing service may be secured to all grades of hospitals, including those for mental diseases, (which we are so apt to leave out of our plans). But as I have already expressed my views on this subject in my paper on

"The Affiliation of Training Schools for Educational Purposes," I need not dwell upon this point.

Nor does our duty cease with looking after our own affairs, for the nature of our work lays upon us heavy responsibilities in relation to humanity. Nurses are peculiarly situated in their opportunities to see life as it really is. From the cradle through all phases of life to the grave, by day and by night, humanity passes through our hands, very dependent, very real, very human. Not even doctors, clergymen or teachers have the same constant opportunity of learning the needs of the people and of judging of the true conditions of life. But it was not during our days of training in the hospitals that these lessons of life were learned, for up to that time our own lives and opportunities had not been different from those about us so that we were not able to read and understand the true significance of sickness and of hospitals. It is only after a nurse has entered upon her work as a graduate, in private duty, in district work, in charge of a hospital, or in taking her share in social movements, that one in whom her work has developed the understanding heart, can look back and read between the lines of her hospital life and know that so much of sickness is preventable and should never have happened, and can realize that health is largely due to the observance of certain and plain fundamental laws, and that sickness is too often only the result of the profound ignorance in mankind particularly among women. Indeed the very number of our hospitals is in one way the proof of the woeful ignorance and neglect that still exist in our social organization. Together with all others interested in the problem of human advancement we are coming to realize that the remedy for this state of ignorance lies in the proper education and development of the child, in opportunities for a broader general education for all and for the special education of all women in matters relating to themselves and personal hygiene, to their home and to their communities, in the equalization and proper adjustment of work, and more particularly of woman's work in the home. Upon the last I would lay special stress because no form of education can be fully effective unless its roots are deep laid in the home and unless women are so educated that they fully realize that home and school life must be drawn close together in such a way that there may be formed a strong, enduring, continuous educational chain that will reach through life. And for this does not the woman need special advantages, and a special preparation? But alas! as things are at present even the ordinary advantages are still lacking, and the only wonder is that women manage to do as well as they do. How long will it be before society realizes that we are daily offering up victims upon the altar of our ignorances. The well being

of the child mentally, morally and physically depends
so much upon the kind of mother or woman that cares
for him that it is almost incomprehensible that from
a selfish standpoint, even putting out of sight one tremendous economic factor in the administration of the
state, we should so long have failed to provide women with suitable advantages to prepare them for
their work in the home. Nor am I speaking of poorer
women only; even those of the favored classes share
equally in the lack of provision of educational facilities for learning the fundamental principles of home
making, of obtaining a practical knowledge of hygiene in its relation to themselves, their children and
their homes and an appreciation of the functions of
the body and the effect upon it of cleanliness, pure
air, food and drink. Parents must understand these
and allied principles and practice them in the home
if the teaching in our schools is to be effective, and
if the world is to be gradually lifted to a higher moral
plane.

When one thinks about these matters it certainly
seems extraordinary that the teachers and leaders in
social reform do not lay more stress upon the importance of the proper education of women. Of
course, lack of proper equipment may be pleaded;
but why not utilize our schools to their full capacity
for various forms of teaching for the parents as well
as the children; and to carry this teaching into fuller

effect why not draw the school and home closer together by making the school the centre for intellectual pursuits and pleasures as well as recreation all the years around, for all in its neighborhood, both young and old? For any education worthy of the name must begin at the cradle and end only with the grave. We must either progress or retrograde, we cannot stand still, and opportunities for progress should be provided for everyone according to his needs, tastes and age. It would not seem impossible to have our neighborhood créches adjuncts to our schools where babies and small children could be left and wisely cared for during hours of recreation, study as well as of work for one or both parents. Nor does it seem impossible that some of the work of the average household which requires the woman of the house to be wife, mother, cook, laundress, nursemaid and seamstress, all in one, should not be centralized and put on a business basis, thus relieving the mother of some part of the heavy daily burdens and affording time for some intellectual life, more recreation, and particularly more time to spend upon the child. Even slight remission from perpetual toil for the mother would certainly be more than compensated for by the higher average of harmony, content and happiness in the home.

Philanthropists have discovered that for juvenile reformatories the cottage plan of school has great ad-

vantages over the congregate plan. They have
further discovered that for juvenile reformatory
schools mental, moral and physical education must
go hand in hand, that equal opportunities must be
afforded for the development of each of that great
trinity of which we are compounded. In the Reformatory School it is found that industrial training makes
for character building, as one writer says it ''tends
to create character by developing the steady hand,
the true eye, working to a plan, obeying orders, conscientious fulfilment of design, steadfast application
to a task, delight in a perfect and finished job, respect for a master who knowns how to plan and produce results, taste for industrial labor, and last but
not least, discovery of one's peculiar aptitude.'' One
wonders how long the world will be in finding out
that precisely all these principles may be applied to
children before they qualify for reformatories; that
schools should represent not a preparation for life,
but life itself, that were more time and thought and
money spent upon the proper development of the
school and home there would be far less need for
juvenile reformatories and for hospitals. People must
have centres to turn to; as it is, the rich man has his
club, the poor man the saloon, or the street corner.
Why should not the school group in a neighborhood
be made the great centre, unsectarian, the common
property of the community, our schools should be the

beauty spots of our towns and country towards which every inhabitant should be able to turn for improvement and pleasure with a sense of personal responsibility and freedom. Such an arrangement would certainly make for a higher citizenship and for a better Christianity.

Next in order should come the development of the home hospital, the neighborhood hospital, for the convenience and comfort of the neighborhood, to be reproduced in our large cities as many times as we have districts. Would it seem heresy on my part to suggest that the day of large hospitals may pass and that in the future they may be superseded by the home hospital? The large hospital has done and is doing good work, but it cannot meet all the needs. One of our vexed questions is how to care for the sick in their homes when they cannot afford the services of a trained nurse, and cannot for various reasons leave their homes to enter the hospital. Furthermore we all know that in a large hospital the flavor of institutionalism cannot be wholly eradicated, nor can the same amount of personal attention be accorded each patient as in the cottage hospital. Would it not be possible to have not only our ward schools but also our home hospital with its staff of nurses, who might be not only the nurses for the sick but also the teachers of health, and thus bring the benefits of the district nurse within the range of all and make her work really constructive and lasting.

Such conditions may sound impracticable but one must see visions and dream dreams before great facts come into existence and some such scheme of education and of living as I have very imperfectly touched upon is no more impossible than were training schools for nurses in hospitals forty years ago. You know that in this matter the impossible was brought about and the change resulted in an entirely different conception of hospitals in the public mind and in a tremendous saving of life. But it required at first women who had the courage of their convictions to meet the strong opposition of families and physicians to prove that it was possible to live through years in such dens of iniquity as hospitals were at that time regarded, and to come out not only unspotted but leaving behind them in these hospital wards an influence by the results of which we are benefitting to-day. This splendid reform was the outcome of the training of the hands, the mind and the heart.

Nurses are unique among women as the first to be provided with this triple form of education, and if it has answered so well in our own case, although still in a state of development, does it not stand to reason that it ought to serve in other forms of work? This training has also given us our definite place and a voice in the work and needs of the community and has carried us beyond the confines of creed and of country, beyond the bounds of luxury and poverty into close communion with the great brotherhood of man. It has opened the door to the higher citizenship; it rests with ourselves whether we shall pass through, and if training has done this for us, is it not our bounden duty to use our efforts to help make it possible for others to bring the home and the municipality into such close relation that one will be the reflection of the other? Can we not help to so educate women that they will realize that the work in the home finds its greater expression in their work in the community? Emerson has said "The reform that applies itself to the household must not be partial. It must correct the whole system of our social living. It must come with plain living and high thinking. It must break up caste and put domestic service on another foundation. It must come in connection with a true acceptance by each man of his vocation, not chosen by his parents or friends, but by his genius with earnestness and love." And to achieve this the foundation stones are the children, every one of whom should in common justice and honesty be given a chance.

Nurses have unlimited opportunities of using their influence by voice, pen and their own lives and work to bring others to a practical realization of the work that must be done through education; and the women in Canada have no ground for shirking their municipal and community responsibilities, for they have free municipal privileges equal to those of the men. They are also fortunate beyond other countries in not having such bad conditions, but with the inevitable growth of the country these must come, unless wisely provided against now. It seems as though with Canada, with her present great opportunities, might rest the solution of the problem of higher citizenship for other countries, but to effect this she must be what she teaches and live as she believes. A political club in Montreal has as its motto, "Every man is individually responsible for just so much evil as his efforts might prevent;" after "Every man" I should like to insert "every woman," and recommend this revised motto as a fitting one for each nurse who wishes to call herself a good citizen.

Titles in This Series

10   Dorothy Deming. *The Practical Nurse*. New York, 1947.

11   Katharine J. Densford & Millard S. Everett. *Ethics for Modern Nurses*. Philadelphia, 1946.

12   Katharine D. DeWitt. *Private Duty Nursing*. Philadelphia, 1917.

13   Janet James, editor. *A Lavinia Dock Reader*.

14   Annette Fiske. *First Fifty Years of the Waltham Training School for Nurses*. New York, 1984. *BOUND WITH* Alfred Worcester. "The Shortage of Nurses—Reminiscences of Alfred Worcester '83." *Harvard Medical Alumni Bulletin 23*, 1949.

15   Virginia Henderson et al. *Nursing Studies Index, 1900–1959*. Philadelphia, 1963, 1966, 1970, 1972.

16   Darlene Clark Hine, editor. *Black Women in Nursing: An Anthology of Historical Sources*.

17   Ellen N. LaMotte. *The Tuberculosis Nurse*. New York, 1915.

18   Barbara Melosh, editor. *American Nurses in Fiction: An Anthology of Short Stories*.

19   Mary Adelaide Nutting. *A Sound Economic Basis for Schools of Nursing*. New York, 1926.

20   Sara E. Parsons. *Nursing Problems and Obligations*. Boston, 1916.

21   Juanita Redmond. *I Served on Bataan*. Philadelphia, 1943.

22   Susan Reverby, editor. *The East Harlem Health Center Demonstration: An Anthology of Pamphlets*.

23   Isabel Hampton Robb. *Educational Standards for
       Nurses*. Cleveland, 1907.

24   Sister M. Theophane Shoemaker. *History of
       Nurse-Midwifery in the United States*.
       Washington, D.C., 1947.

25   Isabel M. Stewart. *Education of Nurses*.
       New York, 1943.

26   Virginia S. Thatcher. *History of Anesthesia with
       Emphasis on the Nurse Specialist*. Philadelphia, 1953.

27   Adah H. Thoms. *Pathfinders—A History of the
       Progress of Colored Graduate Nurses*.
       New York, 1929.

28   Clara S. Weeks-Shaw. *A Text-Book of Nursing for the
       Use of Training Schools, Families, and Private
       Students*. New York, 1885.

29   Writers Program of the WPA in Kansas, compilers.
       Lamps on the Prairie: A History of Nursing in Kansas.
       Topeka, 1942.